CONQUER YOUR FOOD ADDICTION

The Ehrlich 8-Step Program
for Permanent Weight Loss

Caryl Ehrlich

FREE PRESS

New York   London   Toronto   Sydney   Singapore

*f*P

FREE PRESS
A Division of Simon & Schuster
1230 Avenue of the Americas
New York, NY 10020

For information about special discounts for bulk purchases,
please contact Simon & Schuster Special Sales:
1-800-456-6798 or business@simonandschuster.com

Designed by Jan Pisciotta
Illustrations on pages 19, 38, 61, 159, 185,
194, 214, 247, and 248 by Ron Porcelli; copyright Caryl Ehrlich.
Charts by Carolyn Nakano.

Manufactured in the United States of America

1   3   5   7   9   10   8   6   4   2

The Library of Congress has catalogued the Free Press
hardcover edition as follows:
Ehrlich, Caryl.
Conquer your food addiction : the Ehrlich 8-step program
for permanent weight loss / Caryl Ehrlich.
p. cm.
Includes index.
1. Weight loss—Psychological aspects. 2. Compulsive eating.
3. Food habits. I. Title.
RM222.2 .E335 2002
616.85'26—dc21   2002019562

ISBN 0-7432-2974-6
0-7432-3282-8 (Pbk)

I dedicate this book to all who've tried
to conquer the cycle of their food addiction.

Pleasure is not a necessary component of addiction. More plausible is the hypothesis that the addictive element of this behavior is not food, but the cycle itself.

William Ira Benton
Editor, *Harvard Medical Health Letter*

Contents

Dear Reader

This is not a diet book. There are no recipes, no counting of calories or figuring of fat grams. There is no prop or pill, nor is there any diet or deprivation. There is no special food and no liquid concoction to mix. *Conquer Your Food Addiction* is a behavioral approach to weight loss. It is about learning to eat real food in the real world, but it's not even about food. It's about conquering your *inappropriate use* of food.

The weight-weary might be thinking, "But I know what to do." And you might. But if you don't know *how* to do it, you know nothing.

Every opinion, thought, and conclusion about weight loss in this book is my own, gained not only from keeping off 50 pounds for more than a quarter century, but also from successfully teaching my program to thousands of others.

Compulsive overeating is a full-blown addiction because you continue doing what you're doing even though there are negative consequences, and you are in denial about what you're doing and how it contributes to your weight. Even consuming an entire package of TicTacs every day of the year is a weight gain of more than 7½ pounds by year's end.

If you swallowed it, you ate it, and it all adds up.
If it's not water, it's food.

Your ritualized eating behavior is most likely mindless, unconscious, thoughtless, and automatic. My goal is to lead you to mindfulness, consciousness, and thoughtfulness. Instead of thinking, *I'm not doing anything to contribute to my weight problem,* you begin to think: *Oh yes. I do that. Next time, I can do something else.*

You don't change the foods you eat.
You change your habits instead.

Old trigger situations don't disappear. You will feel lonely, tired, bored, frustrated, and angry again. But it's not a reason to eat. You can learn a new automatic response.

This book is designed to help you gently change your thoughts and actions in small, incremental steps from your old *it-isn't-working* way of thinking to a new *can-do-it* way of thinking. Let me hear an *I can do it*. And if you want to learn how it has helped other participants in *The Program,* you can find their verbatim comments throughout the book.

The Program Way

The Program—*everything* I talk about in this book is The Program— begins with a question, one in which most people are interested. What can I eat? they ask. The answer is, Anything; you just can't eat it all in the same meal. The problem is that most people watching their weight are so used to limiting what they can or cannot eat based on the mass of misinformation—ill-informed, over-hyped weight-control messages—in the marketplace that they simply don't get enough variety or satisfaction from what they do eat. The Program shows you more interesting possibilities of how to enjoy what you're eating and still lose weight. Yes, butter on your baked potato is fine.

The more important dimension of this program concerns the inappropriate, ritualized use of food that you've created to distract yourself from feeling things you don't want to feel. It contains many components. Food is just one of them. The other parts are the behavioral ritual blanket you've woven to self-medicate, to zone out; the way your mood, situation, and circumstance dictate when, what, and how much you're going to eat. Before you know it, you're eating just because it's there, or you're bored, or it's the only thing you could find, or the stock market went down (or up). It doesn't matter. You're weaving a ritual web of distraction (from feelings you don't want to feel). That web of distraction comprises the things you say (*I can't eat that; I can't stop once I start; I can't eat in that restaurant*), what you wear (*I only wear dark colors; I can't wear belts; I can't shop in that store; all the clothes in my closet are tight*), finding the right recipes (*This is fat free; this is sugar-free; this is taste free*).

Another part of your web of distraction might be how you buy and keep clothes you've never worn. Or discussing with friends every up and down of how "good" and "bad" you are with your weight-loss plan. Or avoiding going to the beach for fear of walking around in shorts or a bathing suit. When it comes to distracting ritual behavior, it is just as seductive as the smell of a cup of coffee, the texture of a roll, the flavor of a sirloin steak, the crunch of a baked potato. Your behavioral rituals evolved from your parents' passing along to you their family rituals to which you've added some of your own: *This is how I eat in a Chinese restaurant, an Italian restaurant, Sunday brunch, when I celebrate, when I grieve.* These behaviors are familiar and comfortable.

As someone once observed, "It's deadening pain by means of a more intense pain."

Yes. Some idiot might have cut you off on the turnpike. Or a friend hurt your feelings. Or one of your children was sent home from school and you had to leave work early, or you're lonely or tired or angry. No matter. *Eating doesn't change the outcome of anything but your waistline and your self-esteem.*

The mind is ruled by its most dominant thought. If you keep thinking, *This is how and what I eat when I'm depressed,* or *This is how I eat at Passover, at Thanksgiving . . .*, you yield the same old result. You can learn to create something more appropriate for the smaller person you want to be, enjoy the mealtime moment, *and* be happy with the new result.

The Program will lead you from your old way to a new way of thinking and then cheer you on to the finish line as you choose to weigh _____ pounds.

In each segment, you'll read about successful ways that have worked for others. You'll be encouraged to find the method that works for you. The connection between thought, action, and feeling needs to be pulled apart and separated from the ritual of buying, ordering, preparing, serving, and eating food.

If you're hungry, you'll eat. People with diabetes may need to eat differently than The Program suggests. Fourth Meals, explained in the book, will most likely be helpful, but check with your physician to be sure.

Thirsty? You'll drink water. And if neither but thinking about food, you'll learn to create different behavioral rituals to absorb your mind. Any effort is better than none. Perfection is an illusion.

If you stopped smoking or drinking or taking drugs, that would be that. But you can't stop eating, so you have to learn how to do it. The book will show you how best to serve your goal of achieving your desired weight.

The way to deconstruct the snarl of ritualized behavior you've created is to rewrite, in your own handwriting, the foundation of The Program. Then read and reread those sections. Practice the new way, and your new way of thinking and acting will become comfortable, automatic, and preferred.

E-mail your positive stories about The Program to me at: Caryl@ConquerFood.com

And check out my Web site: www.ConquerFood.com

Enjoy the journey.

My Story

I am a compulsive eater. And yet more than twenty years ago, I lost 50 pounds and never gained them back. I didn't wake up one morning and weigh 50 pounds more than I wanted to weigh. It was gradual. Two pounds became 5. Five became 10. And just when I was thrilled it wasn't 15, it became 20, 30, and then 50.

I couldn't wear my rings because my fingers were so fat. Tuck-in blouses were renounced in favor of overtops. A button fell off a pair of pants, but I knew that even if I sewed the button back on, the pants would not fit. The button would not button; the zipper would not zip. In my thirties, I felt like a fat old lady.

I caped and draped to cover my girth and was embarrassed to take off my clothes whether alone or with another. I completely avoided full-length mirrors. I avoided having my photograph taken. I perspired all the time and was frequently out of breath. Eventually, I felt uncomfortable going out at all; I never had anything appropriate to wear anyway.

I once visited my best friend in San Francisco wearing double-digit-size jeans, and they split wide open in the seat. We went to a store where I tried on the largest size pants they carried. I was too big to fit into them. I had to leave the store with my friend's flannel shirt wrapped around my waist so my exposed tush would not show.

For seven years, I suffered with this extra 50 pounds. I didn't want to discuss my problem with friends who count calories or grams of fat. Those friends remained fat. I knew my thin friends didn't know why they were thin. I had been a thin person my entire life, and I didn't have a clue as to why I had been thin. Moreover, I was too ashamed at how out-of-control I was.

I believed the illusion that if I made up my mind to stop eating, I could. But I couldn't. Looking unattractive was bad enough, but it was being out of control that was the scariest. As I was consuming an entire box of cookies, one at a time, I realized I could not stop eating until they were all gone. It was not the first time, and I knew it would not be the last.

It was obvious I had gained a lot of weight. I couldn't fit into my clothes. I was always tired. Yet there was still a modicum of denial, a component of addiction where I continued thinking, "I can handle it," even with so much evidence to the contrary. I'd promise myself that the cookie I was eating was the last, yet I'd eat another. And another. And another. I was in the thrall of food. I used food as a drug, to self-medicate, to zone out, to escape.

I realized that I had many eating rituals like the cookie one. The way I bought and ate certain candy, cookies, or ice cream. The way I'd mindlessly nibble away a box of crackers. The way I'd put something in my mouth whenever I was making a salad. Or how I'd nibble and nosh a leftover until it wasn't left over.

I saw how I *used* food to avoid doing an unpleasant task, to procrastinate, or when I was anxious, or tired, or sad, or angry. I also looked for food before I went out and as soon as I returned home. Food had become a before-, during-, and after-meal activity. It was always one more bite, one more slice, one more sliver. Then I'll feel better. But I never did. All that happened was that I still wanted more.

I purchased and read what seemed like every diet book and magazine ever written on the topic. There were thousands, each with a different angle. There were some where entire food groups were forbidden, as if opting for one food over another would do the trick. One diet recommended frequent servings of meat, including bacon and sausage. Another promoted zero carbohydrates. Some didn't allow Chinese or Italian food. They all said I could never have chocolate again. Nothing covered my real world of working late, restaurant eating, shortage of time, or the persistent stress of daily life.

No one took into consideration who I was as a person. Whether I was 5'2" tall or 5'8". Did I have a husband and child to feed, or was I a single career woman? My personal inclinations or food preferences were not taken into account. Maybe I didn't want lamb chops on Thursday night; maybe I couldn't afford lamb chops. I tried everything, but kept searching.

I went to a fasting farm with a girlfriend. Everyone at the farm gathered around the television set each evening and watched food commercials and exchanged dessert recipes. Many had been coming to the farm for years because when they returned to the real world, they always regained whatever weight they had lost.

My friend and I had been dutiful fasting farm students. We followed the rules, listened to lectures, went to the movies, kept busy, and didn't talk about food. When my friend's mother arrived by car to drive us back to the city, she asked where we wanted to eat our first meal? Though we had not previously discussed it, in unison we cried, "Kentucky Fried Chicken!" So much for a week of abstinence. The few pounds we both lost were regained along with some new extra weight that seemed to creep in every few months.

I must have known that a week of abstinence and deprivation wasn't going to change a thing. It was impractical and unhealthy to skip meals. I wanted to, needed to, learn *how* to eat.

I went to a diet doctor on Central Park South in New York City thinking he had the answer. He did not examine me, take a pulse, or ask for my medical history. Instead, I was given a handful of diet pills and charged for an office visit. When I returned home, I took one pill, stayed up wired for a day and a half, cleaned the apartment twice, and ironed everything in sight. I was contemplating vacuuming Third Avenue when the pill finally wore off.

My frustration and lack of understanding led me to an internist's office where I was given a complete physical and pronounced healthy. When I begged the doctor to tell me what to do to lose weight, he said, "Oh, you know what to do," and sent me home. He was right. I did know *what* to do. I just didn't know *how* to do it. Since the doctor was himself about 40 pounds overweight at the time and I was only 10 pounds overweight, he didn't take my problem seriously.

There's still a sort of universal mind-set of people without this addiction. They think that a little more determination, willpower, and self-control will make a difference. If I could rally it, I thought, why hadn't I done so?

After years of being thin, I couldn't believe that in order to lose weight I would have to deprive myself of foods I enjoy. Did this mean I could never have chocolate again? There had to be a better way.

I was forced to ask questions:

- How do I confront the constant visual blitz of food stimulus?

- How can I feel comfortable with the choices I make in a restaurant when everyone else is eating more and what I perceive to be better food?

- How could I reach my weight loss goal without feeling deprived?

I had also been a smoker and realized that what I learned from stopping smoking could be applied here.

After years of smoking two and a half packs of cigarettes a day, I managed to stop smoking in 1975 without feeling deprived. I had learned that after three to six days, the nicotine is out of your system. All that remains is the ritual habit of smoking; the cigarette with the morning coffee, the cigarette when the phone rings (or doesn't ring), the cigarette after every meal or whenever else I'd feel the slightest bit of anxiety. I was able to stop smoking easily and comfortably by learning how to create constructive new responses to replace the old self-defeating, automatic ones.

Food has no power except the power you give to it by eating in the same ritualistic way, in the same circumstances, for the same inappropriate reasons. If I got into the habit of eating a certain way even though I didn't like the outcome, I reasoned, I could get into the habit of eating another way where I would like the outcome. And if I did it often enough, the new way would be comfortable and the old way something I used to do.

The first steps I took were about awareness.

- To find out how much I weighed, I got on my scale.

- Then I wrote down what I was eating and how often I was eating it. It was the beginning of The Program, on which this book is based.

The next step? The book you are reading. It is the evolution of the solution to conquering your food addiction.

SPEED BUMP

Dave Coverly

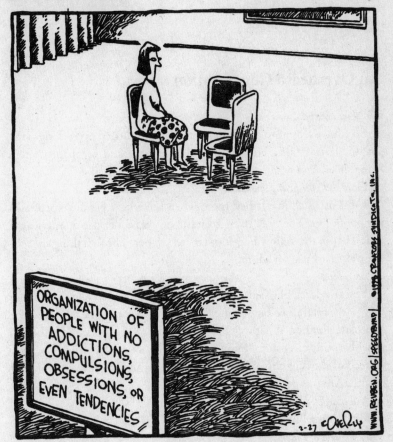

Orientation

An Overheard Conversation

*S*o *then what did you do?*

So I finally went to a weight control lady. I'd tried everything—the spa, the fasting farm, buttermilk and grapefruit, and pregnant woman urine shots! You name it, I tried it. But nothing worked.

How did you hear about her?

I was in a stall in a ladies' room when I overheard two women talking about her. The only thing to write on was toilet paper. Anyway, I found her in the Yellow Pages and met with her. The first thing she told me was that I was an addict.

An addict?

Yes, an addict. She said, "The intelligent me says I shouldn't be doing this"—overeating or bingeing or purging or avoiding fat one week or chocolate another. Whatever I'm doing that I know I shouldn't be doing, I basically can't stop. "Food is my socially acceptable drug," she said. Instead of shoving it up my nose or into my arm, I'm shoving it into my mouth. Are you eating that potato?

No, thanks. Do you want it?

Well. Just a bite.

What else did she say?

I have to keep a log of everything I eat. Get a notebook. Write it all down.

No way.

Exactly. I can't. It's just too humiliating. And of course if I do write it down—and I'm not sure I want to—then I might have to do something about it. Do you want that roll? I just want a bite.

No. You can have it. So are you going to work with her?

I don't know. On the one hand, I want to, have to, must lose some weight. I mean it's not a lot, but I'm so out of control. And she's right: I can't stop once I've started. But I'm not ready to give up all my favorite foods like potato chips or rice pudding with raisins. Of course, she says I don't have to.

Do you want to share some dessert?

Those people over there had something chocolaty. I shouldn't but— well, she said I can have dessert if I'm hungry. But then I have to write it down.

You're going to write it down? I couldn't. I'd be too embarrassed.

She said it was unrealistic to expect to be perfect.

Yeah. But it's still too embarrassing to write it all down.

Let's get the check. It's 11 o'clock, and I have to be up early tomorrow.

No dessert? I had a really bad day, and *dessert always makes me feel better.*

I'll keep you company but none for me. Then I don't have to write down anything.

This weight control lady is a good influence. Okay. Nothing for me either. Let's get the check.

Food for Thought . . .

**In order to have what you don't have,
first you must do what you don't do.**

And then you must do it again, and again, and again, and again, until the new way becomes the comfortable and preferred way.

When you think of a diet, you may be thinking you shouldn't be doing a regime for more than two days, a weekend, a week, ten days, two weeks, a limited period of time.

You might think: Anchovies and buttermilk for ten days? I can do that because *eventually,* I don't have to do that anymore.

A diet has a beginning, a middle, and an end.

The Program is not a diet. To repeat: not a diet, not a diet, not a diet. There is a beginning, a middle, and no end. For whatever reason—genetic, ethnic, hereditary, situational, circumstantial, seasonal, or regional—you've stepped over a line and are eating when you're not hungry. But now and for the future, you might have to think a little differently and plan, buy, prepare, or serve a little differently. No matter what assignments I suggest you do, nothing is as difficult or painful as standing in front of a closet full of clothes that no longer fit. Nothing I tell you is as detrimental to your self-esteem and health as is being so out of control with food.

Whether the mind is creating success or failure, the mind is still creating.

You are a product of your thoughts.

If you continue thinking that you've tried a few things and nothing works, your *Addict Pea Brain*—your reptilian, mindless, unconscious brain—hears that nothing works.

Since the mind achieves its most dominant thought and all you're thinking is that nothing works, that is what you achieve: nothing works.

When you think success, you achieve success.

Think of how you'll look when you reach your weight-loss goal. What do you look like? How do you zip up your skirt or pants? How do you say *yes, thank you,* to offered food? How do you say *no, thank you,* to offered food, when appropriate? How do you look when you walk into a room? Do you blush when someone tells you how great you look?

Think of all the reasons you can do this. It is destructive and serves no purpose to give credence to times when you might not have been as successful as you wanted. Instead think: *What could I do next time?*

"Habit: An acquired behavior pattern *regularly followed* until it has become *almost involuntary.*" *Random House Dictionary*

Think of all the habits you have—the way you brush your teeth, comb your hair, answer the phone, or wash a dish. It doesn't much matter how you wash a dish. Your way is no better than mine and mine no better than yours, as long as the job gets done.

When it comes to eating, however, you've got a habit that is not working for you.

Regularly follow The Program until it becomes *almost involuntary.*

I am willing to change. I choose to change. The choice is mine.

The choice isn't hot fudge or lettuce. You can eat both.

The choice is, Do you want to weigh what you now weigh, or more? (Overeating is a progressive disease. If you knew what to do about your weight, you would have done it 5, 10, 30, 50 pounds ago.) Or do you want to weigh _____ pounds?

Every nanosecond of every minute of every day you have an opportunity to change. The old way is destructive and doesn't feel so good. The new, constructive way does feel good. The choice is yours.

The Ritual of Food Addiction

If you've been trying to figure out the weight-loss game for as long as I've been coaching people (twenty years), you've most likely been trying to avoid food, even though that point of view has not worked. What you need to do is to look at the ritual leading up to the part where you finish everything on your plate.

For many years, I had either a radio show or a public access television cable show named *Changing Habits*. The opening of both shows state: "We cover eating, smoking, gambling, drinking, shopping, spending, and negative thinking." There was also discussion about low-wage earning, debt accumulation, messy apartments, and procrastination. All of these things have something in common: they can be ritualized.

I, too, was seduced by the mesmerizing effect I felt when I was in the mindless, automatic state of a ritual. When in that state of mind, you're comfortable without having to think or feel anything else. I smoked cigarettes, spent too much, drank too much, and went into debt as if I were in a trance. Writing this book became a behavioral ritual; there was always another chapter to write or rewrite or edit or type. I'm in the middle of construction in my apartment. What began as redoing a bathroom and kitchen floor has turned into buying new furniture and designing built-ins.

One tiny part of the redecorating process was looking for knobs for cabinet doors. There were hundreds of styles, shapes, colors, and prices from which to choose. I don't even want to tell you how many choices I had to make when it came to selecting a couch.

Whether gambling or drugging or eating, or writing a book, there is a ritual of things we do, and say, and think, before, during, and after the actual using of the drug. And I use the word *drug* here because a behavioral ritual is just as much a drug on your system as is food, cigarettes, or alcohol.

The gambler knows the phone number of off-track betting or his or her bookie by heart. A bartender remembers your usual drink. You shop whenever you're bored. The drinker has a favorite drink with a specific amount of ice or mixer or water. He or she might sip the drink rhythmically, with or without others at specific times of the day or week or year, and many people drink only in particular places. It never occurs to me to order alcohol in an Asian restaurant, whereas my friend Tom always orders a beer and my friend Sara orders one large and one small sake when in a Japanese restaurant. Each part of a ritual knits with the other parts to tighten the behavior more and more effectively. Add to your list the way you lock and unlock the door to your home or office, answer your phone, call a friend, get ready for bed, set your hair, or comb your moustache.

When I smoked, there was the buying and smoking of the cigarettes. But there was also my cigarette case collection, a Dunhill lighter, and I used a Lalique ashtray, for goodness sake. I added behaviors to my ritual too: I needed to shop for, and have on hand, lighter fluid for the lighter and extra mouth spray and mouthwash to use after I smoked each cigarette.

The ritual paraphernalia is just as much a part of your eating (or smoking or drinking) habit as the lighting up and inhaling of a cigarette or the swallowing of a bite of food. Each habit has its own ritual actions and reactions.

Think about other rituals and habits you mindlessly perform each day. You brush your teeth, shower, shave, or put on makeup. Checking on mail or retrieving telephone answering machine messages may be a part of your repertoire. I've recently added to my ritual the periodic checking of my e-mail—to see if "I've got mail."

Getting dressed in the morning is ritualized too. You might comb your hair and put on makeup, then put on clothes. Others put their clothes on first, and then comb their hair and put on makeup. I eat breakfast and take my one-a-day, two-a-day, three-a-day vitamins and minerals, and my calcium pills. I even arrange them on a paper plate in four little piles for easy access later. That's a ritual too. That's what we do.

We organize and ritualize, so we can narcotize.

All this busywork distracts you, at least for the moment, from feelings or thoughts with which you don't want to deal.

I've practiced and perfected many constructive rituals in my life. After doing them consistently for many years, they are now automatic and mindless, and they serve my needs. They help make my day run smoothly, like using a pencil when I write in my appointment book. There is comfort in the familiar.

It is the ritual of the first thought or word or action that leads to the next thought or word or action to the next, and the next, and the next. Eventually, you succumb to what you think is the allure of the taste, smell, or even sight of food. But it is really the tail end of a ritual where you might be tired or bored and just used to surrendering to whatever is set before you. Some of us eat as an excuse to take a break or to rest. It is hard to say no because it is all knit together from the first thought of a ritual to the first feelings of remorse. There's always remorse. That's part of the ritual too. This cycle of behavioral ritual needs to be interrupted and unraveled. Identifying these patterns—even acknowledging you have patterns—is a wonderful first step in changing habits.

As you become more aware of your patterns of thought, word, and action, you can begin the process of rearranging or omitting the automatic next steps and create constructive new patterns for yourself. Eventually, you'll learn to be comfortable thinking, saying, and doing something else instead of putting food into your mouth just because it's there.

This unraveling of the ritual of food addiction helps you to make choices so you can become the person you want to be. Sometimes the new way is quite different from what you've accumulated in the way of behavior. Your old way was built over a lifetime of unconscious actions and reactions. You now have the opportunity to create something new and wonderful that better serves your present need to weigh _____ pounds.

Bobby F. danced the *I can go all day without eating, but once I start, I can't stop* tango, a remnant from a previous weight-loss plan.

Since evening activities weren't as stimulating as the daytime ones, he was without things to occupy his mind; old feelings and thoughts bubbled up. With no place to go and no one to talk to, he incorporated going into the kitchen into his usual evening activity of killing time. One trip to the kitchen yielded a piece of candy, another trip yielded a nibble of leftover salad, another trip two grapes. The once- or twice-a-night ritual became more and more frequent. It really took off when he had a phone installed in the kitchen. He found himself sitting on a chair with wheels while speaking on the phone and rolling over to the refrigerator where he'd open the door and window-shop the shelves.

When he worked on breaking that ritual, I had him put a little tick mark on a piece of paper whenever he thought of putting something into his mouth. Between 9 P.M. and midnight, he found himself thinking about food forty-two times—approximately one episode every five minutes!

Forty-two times in three hours he had gotten in the habit of putting something in his mouth even though he wasn't hungry. Forty-two times he nibbled a bite of this and a swallow of that just because he was bored. Whether eating one item or one bite from many items, it all adds up. It doesn't matter if it is salad or soda. You're eating when you're not hungry. If you practice this habit every day of the week, you've got a behavioral addiction that becomes a weight gain. Keep doing the same thing, and it becomes a part of the evening's entertainment. When Bobby moved the phone out of the kitchen, the picture changed. His weight changed. His habits changed. This was just one of many patterns he discovered as a result of being mindful. There were even more to find.

He realized that he always ordered a glass of wine when he took clients to dinner and that each meal ended with a cup of coffee. Every visit to a theater to see a movie seemed to be bonded to eating a bag of popcorn or buying a soda. The buying—I call it a compulsion to purchase—is a ritual too.

When I talked about his patterns with another program participant, she commented that keeping the logbook, in which she enters her daily weights and what she eats, was a ritual. I agreed. Some rituals help us to become mindful of what it is we are doing and enable us to see, in writing, the patterns we've created. Some rituals are better than others.

Barbara J. had difficult times at 4 P.M. each day. It was clear that her desire to eat wasn't about hunger; her lunch was usually only a few hours before. It was connected to her children arriving home from school. When she had to prepare food for them, she mindlessly nibbled on the food herself. She also had a phone in the kitchen and practiced some version of talking on the phone and browsing among the bratwurst. You may be thinking: *But I only pick at the broccoli.* If you're eating when you're not hungry, it doesn't matter what it is. It all adds up.

In an office, an eating ritual might begin at the onset of a coffee wagon bell ringing at 10 A.M. and 3 P.M. Rachel S. told me of a mindless habit she had when she commuted from Manhattan to her home in New Jersey. Every trip, five days a week for a year, she'd eat a candy bar. That one candy bar habit could add up to approximately 20 pounds by year's end.

I used to have a habit of buying a large bottle of fruit juice and would sip it a few swallows at a time (*It's only juice,* I used to think) until all 64 ounces were sipped away and I'd buy another bottle. When I realized how often I repeated this behavior, I began buying juice in individual bottles of 4 ounces each, put the bottles on a different shelf from the top one in the refrigerator. If I didn't see it, I didn't think about it. If I didn't think about it, I didn't drink it. The habit started to collapse on its own. Sometimes changing just one part of a ritual—whether thought, word or action—loosens the entire knot of behavior without much effort. Sometimes it takes more thought. In this case, changing the size of the container did the trick (a physical action). I also thought (mental repatterning, to be discussed later) that I'd gone years without drinking juice so many times during a day and it had always been okay. It could be okay again. You get used to anything.

What are some of your rituals and habits?

Denial

A component of addiction is denial. You might travel from thinking, *I'm okay, I'm okay, I'm okay around food* to *I'm not okay.*

Consistently eating more than you need, even though there are negative consequences, is part of the addiction too.

I am an addict. No matter how many years I practice the new, mindful way of eating, the new habits will always be less substantive than the old habits and patterns I have practiced over a lifetime of mindless eating. The old way will always have more practice, heft, weight, and power than the new way.

From years of pushing the envelope myself—that's what addicts do—I know for sure you don't have willpower or self-control; they were both surgically removed at birth. You can, however, learn to buy a little less, order a little less, prepare and serve a little less. By the time food is presented, you'll eat a little less. Ultimately, you'll weigh a little less.

It is the times that you've gone off The Program by leaving food lying around in a too instant, quick, and available form, you're most likely thinking: *I can handle it* or *One won't hurt.* (That's denial.)

It is not one of anything that causes a weight gain. It is that the old way has a ritual, frequency, and portion size that has been established over a lifetime. And if the item you choose happens to be one of the current foods you use to distract yourself, then it is not one of anything, because you can't stop once you've started. You're gonna eat it 'til it's gone.

Do you believe you should be able to leave junk food lying around your home and office and not eat it? (That's denial.) If you're using a food or beverage to distract yourself from feeling angry, lonely, tired, stressed, and worried and you've received some temporary surcease from your emotional discomfort, why should you stop going into the kitchen to get that food—that distraction? When you get there, you always get what you want: something with which to self-medicate. When you create a new automatic response to replace your old automatic response (repatterning), then when you go to the kitchen, the food isn't there. You'll find something else (less destructive) with which to distract yourself. Eventually, you'll stop going into the kitchen.

When you bury feelings, you bury them alive—and not just the bad ones: pain, sorrow, anger, disappointment, but the good feelings of joy and spontaneity as well.

By not stuffing your feelings down one more time, you finally deal with them (the good, the bad, and the ugly) more directly.

The few moments of comfort you receive from drugging with food are totally disproportionate to the quantity of drugs (food, portion size, and frequency of usage) you need to achieve those few moments. Because you build a tolerance to drugs (you cannot ever get it big enough and you can't get it frequently enough) you're never satisfied.

Taking Responsibility

There are no fat fairies who wrestle you to the ground and pour hot fudge into your mouth. You may be making jokes and excuses but there

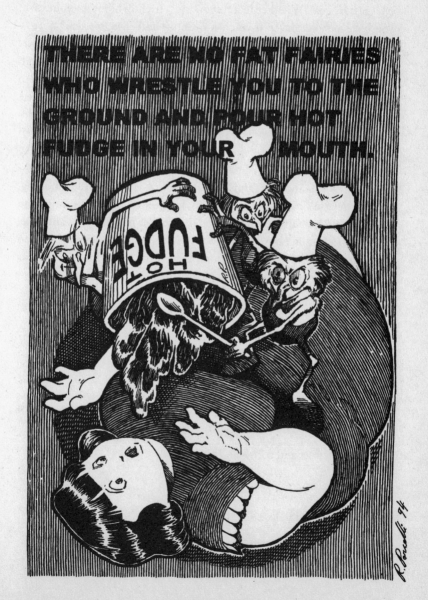

are no demons, comas, or food trances, and the devil didn't make you do it. The culprit is habit.

Every time you shop, order, purchase, and prepare food, there is an opportunity to choose precisely what you want, prepared exactly the way you like it, and more or less in a portion that reflects your ultimate weight-loss goal. Whether in a restaurant, a friend's home, or your own, you have a choice. Even if you are a captive audience, *you don't have to say yes to every course, and you don't have to finish everything on your plate*.

This is no time to lie to yourself. As with changing any other habit, you must honestly define where you are and decide where you want to be. "If you don't know where you're going, you could end up someplace else!" said Yogi Berra. By putting in writing (and in your mind) a detailed plan for what it is you're trying to accomplish, the process of change begins.

There are many types of addictive behavior: eating, smoking, gambling, drinking, and drugging, to name a few. You can stop smoking, gambling, drinking, and taking drugs, but you cannot stop eating. You have to learn how to eat, how to feed the smaller person you want to be.

Even if you don't have an obvious weight problem, you may have an eating behavior that needs attention. Answer the following questions as honestly as possible:

- Do you use food to change your mood?

- Do you need food or drink to add enjoyment to a social situation?

- Do you eat moderately in public or with friends, only to eat in a frenzy when alone?

- Can you go for hours without eating, only to finish an entire basket of bread in a restaurant?

- Do dessert and coffee end every meal?

Why do you want to lose weight?

> "I'm tired of feeling my body plop up and down when I walk."

"I hate standing outside a closet of beautiful clothes while looking for something that will cover my fat. Sometimes I'm not comfortable in whatever I'm wearing."

"I found a bathing suit that I could get into, but I wouldn't parade around any beach looking as I do, so I didn't buy it."

"I stopped skiing because I looked like a stuffed sausage in my ski pants."

It doesn't matter what your reasons are. In order to gain control of your eating, there are areas of responsibility that must be awakened.

Analyze where you are and where you want to be with regard to your weight. Once you have a firm goal, every food choice you make should reflect that goal.

What you weigh. What you weigh, what you eat, and what you're trying to accomplish are the three vital awarenesses. How much did you weigh this morning? How far are you from where you want to be?

Try to be realistic concerning the number of pounds you want to weigh. Set a goal based on the fact that you're not satisfied with your present weight.

Weighing is probably the most resisted assignment. People invest their scale with emotional likes and dislikes, fears and fantasies. Rather than fearing the scale, you should think of it only as the tool it is: to let you know how you're doing. If the number on the scale is on its way down, it is a pleasure to get on it every morning and evening to acknowledge that all your efforts are paying off.

If the needle isn't moving downward, you're most likely continuing to feed the bigger person you were. Maybe you need to slow down when eating. It's not a marathon, it's a meal. If the scale is moving upward, this knowledge will prompt you to take a swift, purposeful, and immediate action so that a 2-pound weight increase won't become 5 and then creep to 10.

Here are examples of how much you weigh in the morning and the evening translates to your weight the next day.

If you weigh 150 pounds in the morning and 152 pounds in the evening, you'll probably weigh 150 pounds the second day:

1st Day	2nd Day
150 A.M.	150 A.M. (no change from previous day)
152 P.M.	

If you weigh 150 pounds in the morning of the first day and 153 pounds that evening, the scale will probably be 151 pounds the second day:

1st Day	2nd Day
150 A.M.	151 A.M. (1 pound weight *gain* from previous morning)
153 P.M.	

But if you weigh 150 pounds the first morning and 151 pounds or less that evening, you'll probably weigh 149 pounds or less the second day:

1st Day	2nd Day
150 A.M.	149 A.M. (1 pound weight *loss* from previous morning)
151 P.M.	

You've burned off almost everything you consumed that day. Your body burned the stored fat. That's what you're striving for: burning stored fat.

What you eat. Keeping a log is another tool you need to help you achieve awareness of your eating habits. Keeping a record of what you eat is a small part of the information you'll garner from a log once you understand you're creating resource material. Your eating is unique, and your log will reflect that fact.

A log will help you to make the connection between what you are eating and what you are weighing. It will point out the foods you choose most frequently and help you identify the times you are most likely to overeat. (Weekends? Holidays? Dinner with friends?) As soon as you enter your home, do you look for something to eat? Do you use food in the afternoon as an excuse to take a rest break? You'll see patterns emerge in your log.

What you are trying to accomplish. Measuring your chest or bust, waist, hips once at the onset of your weight-loss program and once when you reach your goal is an interesting exercise. It shows that you lost inches. For larger people, the ratio is approximately 10 pounds per inch, one belt notch, or suit, shirt, or dress size smaller. For others, even a 5-pound loss could be a smaller clothing size.

As your clothes get looser, you'll realize you're getting smaller. You're losing inches. Be aware that you lose inches all over. You may not be aware you have lost inches in these areas, but your blouse or shirt feels looser, a zipper slides more easily, pants are hanging, and your ring is spinning on your finger.

When I'd gained weight, a ring I frequently wore became so tight I was unable to remove it from my pudgy fingers even with soap and water. A jeweler had to cut the ring off my finger.

Food preparation. I asked a man in one of the sessions who was responsible for food preparation in his home. He said impishly, "I don't know how responsible I am, but I do it."

Taking responsibility isn't only selecting the correct foods. It is learning how to plan ahead and shop a little differently, buy a little differently, and prepare, serve, and eat differently.

Planning the foods you will eat with an eye on the day's activities is being responsible, as is deciding on foods with the best balance, variety, and overall nutrition. Think about which category of food (protein? soup? salad?) you're planning to eat if you hadn't had that same category already today. Or yesterday at the same meal.

Saying no. Being responsible is finding the right words to head off others when they insist on offering food and won't take no for an answer. It is declining the waiter's offer of a second piece of bread, choosing a glass of wine rather than sharing a bottle, or eating only when *you're* hungry, not when others are. Being responsible is creating an atmosphere in which you make the right choices with confidence, once the right choices are acknowledged. Only you can say no.

Alternate activity. Learning to breathe deeply is a responsible day-to-day practice. It supplies oxygen to the brain and helps burn fat the way aerobic exercise increases oxygen to the brain. Relaxing helps reduce stress, lessens anxiety, and becomes a healthful replacement for many discomforts. To delay and eliminate your old automatic response of, "I want what I want when I want it," inhale deeply through the nose, hold to the count of five, and exhale slowly while relaxing body parts from head to toe.

Mouth freshening. Taking responsibility is making sure you always have a toothbrush and tube of toothpaste in your pocket or purse, at the office or in a restaurant, where mouth freshening may be the right move away from the food table. (Sometimes people don't feel like eating with the taste of toothpaste in their mouths.) Valerie and I laughed (another wonderful repatterning technique) when she thought I'd suggested brushing her teeth while she was sitting at the dinner table. Of course, what I meant was for her to excuse herself from the table to brush her teeth in the ladies' room of the restaurant.

Drinking water. Eight to ten glasses a day are essential. Carry water wherever you go. Put bottled water in the car along with plastic cups. Take it on a plane or train when traveling, as well as to the movies. Ask a waitperson to leave a pitcher on the table in a restaurant, and drink a glass or two before eating.

As I'm typing this chapter, there is a bottle of water next to my computer. Is there a bottle of water near you while you're reading this chapter? No? Get some.

Being responsible is not becoming cocky, complacent, or comfortable while losing weight, or after your goal is reached. If you've created new habits while attaining your goal, being responsible is to avoid thinking, "I don't have to do this any more."

Food is available everywhere you go. You will encounter numerous occasions each day where there are eating opportunities. Each time you encounter a fork in the road, you have the choice of going in either direction. The old choice may feel comfortable. It *is* familiar, but it has an unhappy result. A new choice may feel awkward and unfamiliar at first but presents the real possibility of reaching your weight-loss goal. As you consider your choices, repeat over and over to yourself: I want to weigh _____ pounds. Envision a slimmer, confident, more attractive person—an improved version of the present you. Imagine in detail the terrain you're going to travel each day, the foods you are going to eat, whether to have a *Filler* (by the end of the book you'll know what that means), the number of items you're going to eat, and the alternative behavior that may prove successful if your Plan A isn't working. The entire process can be considered in a minute or two . . . as when you're traveling in a car and give thought to which route is best. Do the same by thinking about the best path to follow with your eating habits.

If a difficult moment arises before, during, or after a meal, ask yourself these questions:

> Was I thinking of eating two minutes before I saw food?
>
> Will this food help me reach my weight goal?
>
> Am I even hungry?

Write a paragraph or two about why you want to weigh _____ pounds (not why you don't want to weigh your present weight).

An example might be, "I, _____ [insert your full name], want to weigh _____ pounds [insert your goal weight. Go for it!], because:"

_____

_____

Give thought to the reasons you want to weigh _____ pounds. You may want to look better and feel better, fit more easily into your clothes. Perhaps you want to have high energy and higher self-esteem. Think about how you will look and feel when you reach your goal.

If you want these things, it means you not only don't have them, you most likely have the reverse. You may be unhappy, out of breath, not fitting into your clothes, feeling unsexy, have low self-esteem, and no energy. *That is the cost of your addiction.* Now write those paragraphs.

Unrealistic Expectations Can Cause Failure

Weight gain is an evolutionary process. Some people call it creeping weight. The scale turtles inexorably upward—a tight skirt, a belt notch, a can't-zip-up-my-pants inch at a time. Yet you expect the scale to go down as rapidly as a high-speed elevator. This erroneous thought pattern—practiced and perfected as with any other bad habit—is an unrealistic expectation. It is dangerous with any endeavor and deadly when it comes to weight reduction.

I could have, I should have, I didn't, I wanted to are the loud laments of the perfectionist. Perfection is an illusion, however. Since you'll never be perfect, in your mind, you don't ever succeed. Then you think: *I failed, I blew it, I'm weak* (or bad), or whatever you say to beat yourself up, and you stop trying altogether.

Why not acknowledge small, incremental improvements—times when you did better at one meal, one day, or one event than you might have? Focus only on what you did, not on what you thought you should have done. The inclination to focus on the negative is part of the all-or-nothing addict mind. You think that if you can't do it perfectly for an entire week (even though it is unrealistic to think you can), you won't do it at all. It would be more pleasurable to look for the positive and see that list grow.

All-or-nothing thinking is far more destructive to your weight-loss goal than a friend baking brownies and leaving them on your desk. If you eat even one brownie but manage to give the rest to coworkers and friends, you think you've blown it. A better way of thinking would be to realize you ate only one, when in the past you probably would have eaten several, or maybe all.

Unrealistic expectations give substance, heft, and power to an unrealized goal. They quash the budding crocus of success as it pushes through the thick asphalt of failure. Unrealistic expectations kill the flowering of dreams, because you become so disappointed that you give up hope.

Thomas Edison never stopped trying. "I have not failed 10,000 times," he said. "I have successfully found 10,000 ways that will not work."

The only reality is where you are today—perhaps 150 pounds—and where you were a week ago—perhaps 155 pounds. And even if your weight remains the same, there are other questions to ask: Did you keep a food log of everything you ate? Did you drink the requisite amount of water? Did you do better with your eating at an industry function than you might have? Did you eat less than usual at your mother's? Yes? Then you're ahead of the game.

Marcia S., an unrealistic thinker, lost 7 pounds in two weeks. The third week she lost 1 pound. When I asked for a positive story, she said, "Nothing good happened." She was miserable.

"But you lost 8 pounds," I reminded her.

"Yeah, but," she continued, "I was so good all week, and the scale didn't move."

"You lost 1 pound this week," I reminded her, "and you didn't gain back the previous 7."

"Yeah but . . . " she repeated. "I lost that pound at the beginning of the week and didn't lose anything the rest of the week." She was unable to acknowledge anything positive. So great were her unrealistic expectations that it was impossible for her to feel joy or satisfaction in what she had accomplished.

Ignoring these fragile buds—by not watering, nurturing, and turning them to sunlight—they turn to dust. You're used to seeking out the imperfect, and because you're not yet in the habit of recognizing the fruits of your labor, they dwindle on the vine. What remains are the weeds of destructive, negative, unrealistic thinking. These thoughts can and do take over your mind and your heart. Unrealistic expectations make you believe you'll never succeed, every effort is for naught, and you are forever destined to fail.

If you give too much credence to your real or imagined failures and not enough to your attempts, your interim successes, and your accomplishments, you will become the failure you think you are.

Were your parents critical and judgmental? Are you too hard on yourself? You may have internalized their voice.

Create your own positive voice. Think of the reasons you want to

Fantasy: Some people believe others travel from A to Z on a straight weight-loss path.

Reality: All people travel from A to Z by stopping off at B through Y.

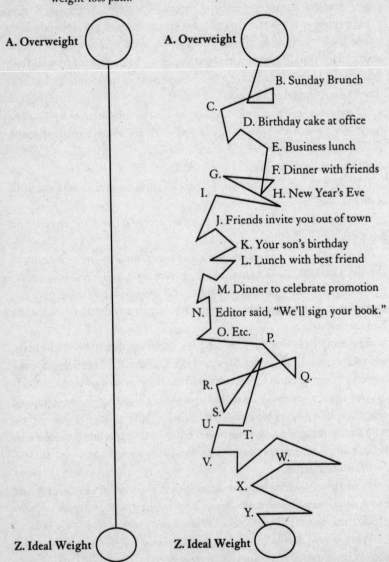

A. Overweight

A. Overweight

B. Sunday Brunch

C.

D. Birthday cake at office

E. Business lunch

G.

F. Dinner with friends

I.

H. New Year's Eve

J. Friends invite you out of town

K. Your son's birthday

L. Lunch with best friend

M. Dinner to celebrate promotion

N. Editor said, "We'll sign your book."

O. Etc.   P.

Q.

R.

S.

U.

T.

V.   W.

X.

Y.

Z. Ideal Weight

Z. Ideal Weight

Hopefully, you'll learn from each stumble and think about what you could do *next time*. There's *always* a next time.

reach your weight-loss goal (or any other goal), not the reasons you don't want to remain at your present weight.

Tell friends how good you feel rather than reliving your less-than perfect efforts. Give importance to the good stuff. Let everything else go.

Try to monitor your negative, unrealistic thinking. See how many times you give yourself credit for doing something positive—"I only ate when I was hungry the entire week"—only to take it away by adding, "... except for Thursday night when I worked late and had three slices of pizza." It is not a good habit of thought to give one evening of pizza the same weight as six days of staying on your program.

Thinking realistically and positively may be tricky at the beginning because you've been thinking unrealistically and negatively for a long time. It takes practice and perseverance to change your attitude, but you will succeed. Perhaps not immediately. Perhaps one baby-step at a time. Perhaps 10,000 attempts later. But, as Georgia O'Keeffe said, "You musn't even think you won't succeed."

Misdirected Anger

Maryanne C., a jogger, broke her ankle while getting off a bus. There was no one to blame for the accident, yet Maryanne blamed herself. "I should have watched where I put my foot," she said. "I wasn't holding onto the railing tight enough. I learned my lesson." She then went home and made herself feel better, with food.

Oh, yeah. That'll do it. Eat. Gain weight. Put more pressure on the al-ready strained limb. I can't imagine why the doctor didn't think of that.

Maryanne's injury hurt physically, but she was in even more emo-tional pain from feeling stupid about her accident.

When she went to dinner with friends, she ate twice as much as everyone else. When she got home later, she ate the leftovers she'd brought home for tomorrow's lunch.

In a short time, the feel-better food didn't feel so good: she'd gained back some of the weight she had lost. She also felt depressed. She was out of control with food again but couldn't seem to stop eating.

If you're eating because you're angry instead of hungry, you're using food to stuff down feelings, not to nourish your body.

Unvented anger becomes like gasses in a pressure cooker. Stuffing down feelings such as anger does not allow them to be examined. Eventually, the feelings build up and finally explode into misdirected action, hurting yourself by eating when you're not hungry. You might think that the way to make anger go away is to stuff it down with food, to self-medicate, to zone out the brain, to narcotize. But when you bury feelings, you bury them alive. This type of behavior doesn't resolve anything. You eat, and you gain weight. You gain weight, and you get depressed. You get depressed, and you eat again—but you're most likely still lonely, tired, bored, frustrated or angry, and you *still* have your weight problem.

To stop the cycle of addiction, try to identify the original feelings of pain to release the long-pent-up feelings. Try to make a connection by asking yourself questions such as, "Does this incident remind me of anything in my childhood?" Or, "Does this person remind me of anyone in my childhood?" If you're self-medicating with food, it is hard to feel. One woman finally realized this truth when she said, "Oh, I see. I don't always have to make myself feel better. I just have to make myself feel."

Try keeping a feelings journal. Instead of letting thoughts and feelings spiral into an out-of-control eating episode, write. As you do this, you'll be able to identify the moments when you're thinking of eating. Ask yourself: "Am I hungry, or what?" The answer might be: "Hungry? How could I be hungry? I just ate an hour ago."

By writing, you'll discover that the things that cause you psychological pain today were most likely learned in childhood. The urge to use food to quell these feelings—to literally stuff down sadness or anger, for example—begins at an early age too. Sometimes you're in denial until you hear someone else's story and realize you do that too.

Lynn P. was losing weight, although she continued to eat almost every night *after* dinner. It didn't seem like much: a bowl of cereal at 10:00 P.M., leftover chicken from the night before, a handful of grapes, and so on. I told her that although she was losing weight and would most likely reach her goal weight, if she continued *eating after eating,* she would not be able to keep off the lost weight because the need to use the drug would increase in volume and frequency. It's progressive.

I suggested she use writing as a repatterning technique in lieu of eating. She should pick two days during the week and one on the weekend when she would not eat after dinner. In all three instances, she would write instead of eat.

She told me later how this worked: "I didn't eat after dinner on Tuesday or Sunday as planned. I didn't use any repatterning techniques to get me through the difficult time. I said I wouldn't eat, and I didn't. I just came home, got ready for bed, and used my up-until-now nonexistent willpower and self-control to get through the next few hours." She called me after each episode, and I told her that toughing it out has a limited effect because the next time, you'll be a little more lonely, tired, bored, frustrated, or angry, and you will eat. I urged her to write about feelings the following Monday—after dinner with friends.

She later told me that she had done this: "I put pen to paper, and for the first ten or fifteen minutes I wrote things like, 'I hate Caryl' or 'This is the stupidest thing I've ever done,' but then something interesting happened. I began writing about my childhood and my mother, and I did that for about fifteen minutes. It just kept pouring out of me—the sadness I felt when my mother would leave every evening for dinner or the theater. I always felt abandoned. And then I began to cry . . . really big crocodile tears. I couldn't stop sobbing and crying, but I kept writing, and the crying continued for almost a half-hour. It was the first time this ever happened except years ago when I was in therapy, but when it was over, I dried my eyes, turned on the television, and read the newspaper until I fell asleep. I had no desire to eat."

I'd be lying to you if I claimed that Lynn never had the urge to eat after eating again. She continues to have these urges, but now she diffuses them more quickly than ever before. She writes in her journal or brushes her teeth or calls a friend. She also understands the connection between her feelings and her inappropriate food usage. And since she knows the writing exercise has worked several times, it will work again and again. In that way, her new automatic response (to write and feel) has replaced her old automatic response (to eat and not feel).

Try this exercise. You'd be surprised at what floats to the top once you've abstained from your drug, food.

Talk to yourself. Are you alone? Did friends just leave? Perhaps you're reliving childhood fears of abandonment.

Did you just get cut off by another driver, another speaker? You may be angry at not being able to express your feelings.

Is a coworker too busy to listen to your problems? Maybe you're feeling lonely or angry. After all, you listened to her when she had a problem. Try to understand it. You learned these conditioned responses in childhood.

Perhaps the driver reminds you of a cousin who drove recklessly, or the coworker too busy to listen to your problems might remind you of a childhood relationship with an older sibling who was always too busy to give you any attention. You might be stuck in that childhood trauma. It might seem foolish to be thinking about it as an adult, but that doesn't mean it isn't a valid connection. You certainly could enter short-term therapy, but unless you're completely immobilized by your behavior, try to make some of these connections yourself.

Do you find yourself eating cookies late at night and convince yourself you're there because it tastes good? If you clean your cabinets of all these [instant/require no preparation/easily available] foods and you find your hand in the breakfast cereal box, you know it's not because it tastes good. Try to repattern by dealing more directly with the feelings. Eating when you're not hungry only changes the measurement of your waistline and further erodes your self-esteem.

Repatterning is delaying an instant (and temporary) gratification. It gives you insights into your eating disorder. Often waiting, even a few minutes, helps one more moment pass without eating. You experience a catharsis in expressing the emotions you've only stuffed down with food in the past. You'll experience a proud sense of accomplishment at making a great plan, executing it, and ultimately peace of mind in understanding the inappropriate way you've been using food.

I saw Lynn the day before New Year's Eve. She'd planned a party for a few family members and close friends. "It's going to be dessert and champagne, but I've also made a pot of pea soup for me and those who might want something to cushion the alcohol," she smiled, clearly pleased with her pre-party planning. As we walked into her kitchen, she showed me all the plastic containers and plastic bags waiting on the countertop for guests who'll be taking home leftovers, a wonderful example of repatterning thought, action, and outcome.

I Speak to You One-on-One

Let's think of each of the following chapters as a session, in which I speak to you one-on-one.

The pages that are marked for you to rewrite into your own logbook are the same forms participants in The Program are told to rewrite when they meet with me. Rewriting will help you internalize the information. You will know that you are internalizing the information when you start using the terms you've found in the book.

The other information in the book is everything I would have said to a participant had we had more time to spend together. These are the things I would say if I could speak to each one of you in person when you work on patterns newly identified as time goes by.

And so I've thought of these chapters as sessions, in which you're meeting with yourself daily or more often. In that way, you will progress as slowly or quickly as you are able. I recommend approximately a seven-day interval between the reading (and filling in) of the review and assignments for each session. This will give the information time to take hold. Practice each week's assignments until they are reasonably internalized. Then you will be ready to handle the next layer of program concepts.

Since each week's assignments build on the previous week's assignments, repetition and review are important so you will be reminded of the things that need to be done—need to be *practiced. The smallest insight, when repeated daily or even weekly, can make the biggest difference in your weight.*

The Basics

What Is Real Hunger?

In order to identify hunger, you must first understand what it is, and this is not as easy as it seems. Many of you may never have let yourself experience true hunger, only a feeling of discomfort. Not knowing exactly what it was, you may have been eating past hunger for such a long time you can no longer differentiate between hunger and the feeling of anxiety, stress, boredom, or any number of other emotional or circumstantial stimuli. You haven't allowed yourself to go without eating for a long enough period of time to have felt true hunger; you may not have experienced it since childhood.

Each of us is born with an innate sense of hunger. When you were a baby and felt this sensation, you cried. Your mother or caregiver pacified you with a bottle or breast, and when you were no longer hungry, you pushed the food away. Before you could speak, you made yourself understood.

As a toddler beginning to eat baby food, you were still in control of your food consumption. Your mother might have thought you had to finish everything she served, but you had other ideas. You might have clenched your little baby teeth and not permitted one extra spoonful of anything to enter your mouth. She might have pushed your chubby little cheeks together trying to force you to open your mouth, but you would not. If she did manage to insert some food, you spit it out (sometimes on your bib, sometimes on Mom.) The message was clear: "No more food, Mommy."

As she persevered, you finally learned to please your mother by finishing everything on your plate. You may have been told that if you ate your vegetables, your reward would be dessert. You were bribed with a lollipop if you'd stop crying. You learned to eat all your food because it gave pleasure to others. It didn't seem to matter anymore whether you were hungry. You were taught to ignore your feelings of hunger and satiation just to please someone else, and you learned well.

Years later, you're still keeping a friend company by sharing a meal

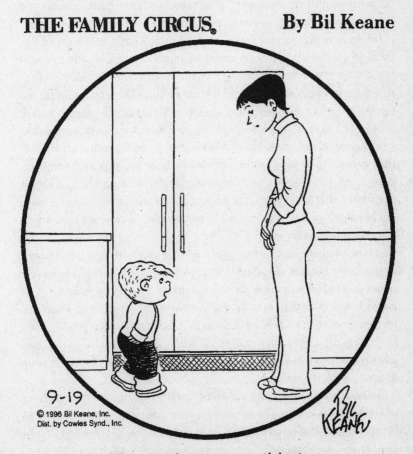

THE FAMILY CIRCUS.   By Bil Keane

9-19

© 1996 Bil Keane, Inc.
Dist. by Cowles Synd., Inc.

"I'm not hungry, or thirsty,
or any of that stuff. What I'd
REALLY like is a hug."

when you're not hungry or accepting an alcoholic beverage just to be part of the crowd or to please a hostess.

The dictionary describes hunger as "the painful sensation or state of weakness caused by need of food." Some people become irritable, shaky, or disoriented if they are not fed at their usual mealtime. Others experience hunger as feeling lightheaded, empty, low, headachy, or hollow. At times, a growling stomach prompts an eating episode. Some eat when they get depressed. Others lose their appetite when they get depressed. External stimuli are abundant, as are emotional and physical ones, yet few of these are hunger—just some other strain on your nervous system.

Human beings have a built-in fight-or-flight mechanism that helps them to survive. When your ancestors roamed the earth and encountered a tiger who had leaped out of the bushes, they would mobilize themselves to fight the tiger or flee from it. Years later, you still face the tigers. A death in the family, loss of a job, or an illness may certainly have the bite of a tiger. Your pulse quickens, your mouth feels dry, your palms sweat, and you revert to old behavior and try to quell the anxiety by putting something in your mouth. You also may be reacting to the fluctuations of daily life—a waiter being inept, traffic inching along, a line at the bank—that cause you to eat a box of cookies or ask for a second helping of food. You might be misidentifying a minor travail as a tiger when it is only a baby cub.

Have you had the experience of thinking you were hungry at noontime, only to become absorbed in a project or in a book and have several hours pass before you think about food again? True hunger cannot wait a few hours; it demands to be fed. You were not hungry at noon but were responding to a time-of-day stimulus, another reason you've given yourself to eat. If you distract yourself with some other activity, the urge usually passes within a few minutes. Try to differentiate between your *hungers* and your *urges*.

Food need not fill you up in order for you to feel satisfied. A few bites of foods you don't usually eat can be very satisfying, while baskets of bread, mugs of coffee, or liter bottles of diet soda might leave you feeling hungry and unsatisfied.

It is *not okay* to eat when you are physically or emotionally uncomfortable. Eat when you're hungry. Stop eating when you are *no longer hungry,* not when you are full or there is nothing remaining on your plate. As your clothes get looser, you'll start to enjoy leaving food on your plate. It is a process that takes time to achieve. Remember:

- *Volume* of nonnutritious food merely stuffs and bloats but does not satisfy real hunger.

- *Variety* and texture, along with nutrition, satiate hunger.

What Does Hunger Feel Like?

To get reacquainted with the true feeling of hunger, try the following exercises:

1. Choose a day when you don't have a specific time or place to eat lunch—perhaps a Saturday or Sunday.

2. Create a relaxing, pleasurable 20-minute breakfast consisting of wonderful hot cereal that takes at least 5 minutes to cook (*not* an instant packet). Season it with whatever will make it most enjoyable for you.

3. After you eat, create a day full of pleasurable food-free activities. Indulge in a massage, a movie, or a late-afternoon nap; write a long-overdue letter; take a day trip to a nearby city or state. Choose things that you find enjoyable—things that will draw on your intellect.

4. After each activity, relax for a few minutes before going on to the next.

5. If possible, avoid clocks, which may be reminders to eat just because of the hour.

6. When you finally believe you're hungry, ask yourself these questions:

   - What is this feeling? Is it hunger? Is it anxiety?

   - How do my head, face, shoulders, chest, stomach, arms, and legs feel?

   - Did something I saw or smell trigger my hunger button?

- Am I thinking of food because I'm tired or bored?

- Am I thinking of eating just to get it out of the way?

- If I don't eat now, will I find time later?

- Did someone else suggest that I stop for lunch?

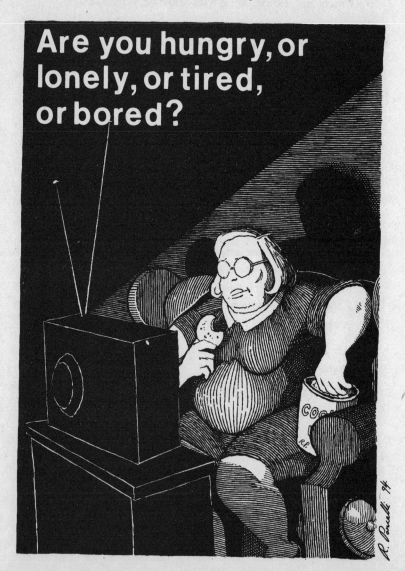

Are you hungry, or lonely, or tired, or bored?

- Am I saying yes to food because someone else wanted to eat?

- Is sitting down to eat an excuse to get off my feet?

Try to get in touch with the total feeling—the true meaning—of why you're thinking about food, why you believe you're hungry. When you can do this—and it might be some time before you can do it with certainty and regularity—you will know whether the feeling is really stress, anger, tension, fatigue, or real hunger.

How many hours passed between eating your hot breakfast cereal and your first bite of lunch? If a bowl of cereal gives you approximately 6 hours of food and energy even if you have not eaten for 12 hours (from a 7:00 P.M. dinner the night before to a 7:00 A.M. breakfast), you realize that your lunch need not contain more food aggregately than the bowl of cereal you had a few hours earlier for breakfast.

How many bites of food did it take before you felt not so hungry? How many of the 20 minutes passed before you felt comfortable?

7. Before consuming any food, ask this question: Am I hungry enough to create a relaxing, pleasant meal lasting at least 20 minutes or more, consisting of food on a plate to be eaten with utensils?

If the answer is yes, create that relaxing, pleasant meal. Once you identify hunger, then when you're feeling another discomfort, you'll think, *That's not hunger because now I know what hunger feels like. That's frustration or anxiety or sadness or joy.* If the answer to "Am I hungry?" is no, continue to repattern until you can identify with certainty the feeling as hunger. When that finally happens, welcome it home!

Possible Pitfalls

There are as many reasons you've given yourself to eat as there are minutes in a day. Storm clouds do it for me. They trigger a memory from when I lived in Florida and went deep-sea fishing in Key West. When a squall was imminent, we'd pull our boat into a nearby atoll and wait out the storm while eating fresh fish sandwiches and drinking cold beer. Sandwiches are finger foods, which I now steer clear of, and I don't drink beer anymore, but the smell of a rainstorm can be a powerful pitfall for me. I don't act on it, but the memory is a tantalizing trigger nevertheless.

A splash of red wine on white pants may not trigger an overeating episode nor will the car not starting, a flat tire, and your cell phone losing a signal at 4:58 P.M. when you must reach someone before 5:00 P.M. But these things have a cumulative effect, and all the mini-annoyances have the potential of becoming maxi-eating responses by the end of the day.

You might stumble because you saw your favorite dessert on a restaurant menu, or a celebration may convert a tentative *no* to an emphatic *yes* as soon as you hear a champagne cork pop from a bottle.

"I can resist anything but temptation," said Oscar Wilde.

Highlight or circle the reasons to which you respond. Consider the following possible pitfalls, reasons people are tempted to eat. There are many, and they are varied.

Do you eat because you're hungry—or because you're lonely, tired, angry, or bored?

Think of all the reasons you eat that have nothing to do with hunger.

Perhaps you eat because you're up: it's your birthday, my birthday, our anniversary, or Groundhog Day—or because you're down: sad or grieving. You might eat because food is there, or someone else is eating, so why not you? Is food easily available in your office or your home? Do you eat in your car?

Are you eating because of good news? Bad news? No news? One man said he eats *during* the news.

You might find yourself eating some foods because they came with a restaurant dinner or others because they came free with your airplane ticket or hotel room. There's bread on the table in a restaurant, peanuts on the plane, chocolates on your pillow, and you think: I'll never pass this way again.

To some, food is a reward: *I've been so good all day. I didn't have breakfast. I didn't have lunch. I'll just have this side of beef for dinner.* Of course, if you're feeling stuffed, bloated, and not so good about yourself, then overeating is not a reward. It is a punishment.

When a young woman used the excuse that she overate prior to going to the ballet, I asked, Did you dance? Unless she was dancing on that stage, she ate too much for dinner. She ate more than she was able to burn.

For many, food has become a socially acceptable drug. It seems to numb the tensions and stresses of life. Perhaps you use food to stuff down feelings and thoughts you don't want to feel or think or to escape.

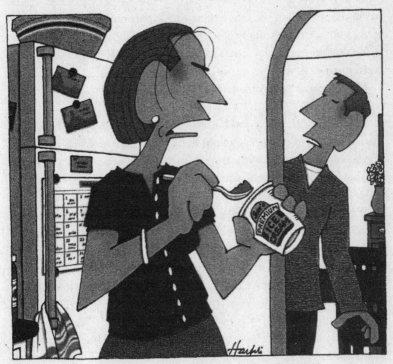

"I'm not eating. I'm self-medicating."

Do you eat when you're frustrated, disappointed, or angry? One fellow told me he knocked off a box of cookies and a pint of ice cream when the court awarded his ex-wife a big divorce settlement. I wanted to know if she had returned the alimony check when she realized he was hurting himself.

Although eating doesn't change the outcome of anything but your waistline and self-esteem, you might still be eating to cheer yourself up when you're down. Or not to feel so alone when you're without company. Or to socialize: you don't want to be left out. You might continue eating even though your clothes are too tight and you're huffing and puffing when you walk. That is part of addiction: *you continue doing what you do even though there are negative consequences.*

Perhaps you eat because you're bored or have to fill unstructured time, such as evenings and weekends, or because you experience family, business, money, or peer group pressure ("Come on. We're all going for pizza, and, we want you to come.") You don't want to be left out.

You might use food to avoid intimacy or sex. Perhaps you use food to avoid nurturing or being nurtured.

Maybe you are procrastinating ("I'll have lunch first and then work on that report").

You might eat during food preparation and put-away. Perhaps once you start, you can't stop. You might think, *What the hell, I blew it anyway.* Maybe you use food as a reward because you did something wonderful or as a punishment because you already overate and figure, *What the hell, it won't make a difference.*

When you smell the coffee in your office, or the popcorn in a movie, or fresh doughnuts in a bakery, do you queue up? Do you use food as a meal extender? You're having such a nice time and don't want the evening to end, so you order another cup of coffee, a cocktail, a dessert. You're entertaining guests. There is an abundance of extra food and all those leftovers.

Going home to family is tricky for some. You may feel guilty that your family and friends have been cooking since last Thursday, and you have to taste (and comment on) everything that is offered. Does the cook get offended if you don't have seconds and thirds?

We eat differently when we are in the company of two people, three people, four people, more people. A recent study said that people who eat with six or more other people consume a whopping 78 percent more than they would if they ate alone. The more people there are, the more food is offered. And the longer food remains on the table, the longer you're tempted to eat.

Are you too tired to cook so you *pick pick pick* and convince yourself you didn't eat anything?

A point to remember:

If you swallowed it, you ate it. It all adds up.

And this, too:

If it's not water, it's food.

Whether you overeat because of genetics, ethnicity, religion, circumstance, or emotion doesn't matter. Perhaps you eat for some of these reasons or all of these reasons. Each person gets into the habit of using food inappropriately by eating for reasons you tell yourself it's okay to eat, even if you're not hungry. Having followed these habits for such a long time—sometimes decades—they've become involuntary conditioned responses. Just like Pavlov's dogs, when a stimulus appears, can a *yes, thank you,* be far behind? The intelligent you thinks you shouldn't be doing what you're doing, but you can't stop. That's the sneaky part of the addiction—as if making up your mind will do the trick when it never has before. This might be the moment to make a list of the reasons *you* eat. Put down the breadstick and get a pencil.

After seeing my list, a middle-aged woman said to me, "According to your program, I haven't been hungry since 1963." She was correct. She and you may have misidentified these situations, circumstances, and emotions as hunger for such a long time that you've lost your innate ability to identify this most basic of feelings.

If you're trying to satisfy a physical hunger, your body doesn't require a great deal of food. If you're trying to fill an emotional hunger, you could back up a truck full of food to your home or office, and it would never, ever contain enough food. "Okay, guys, put the Mallomars in the cabinet, the Häagen-Dazs in the freezer. The Twinkerdoodles go on the bed."

If you become so overwhelmed, confused, and paralyzed with not knowing what to do about this multifaceted, many-layered topic of weight control that you can't stop eating once you start, chances are you do nothing.

If hungry, you need to nourish the body. If it also tastes good, looks good, and smells good, you've got a bonus. But you shouldn't be eating *because* it looks, smells, and tastes good. Almost everything fits that criterion.

If you're thirsty, drink water.

If you're responding to one of the above stimuli, change habits by cre-

Person Filled with Excuses to Eat

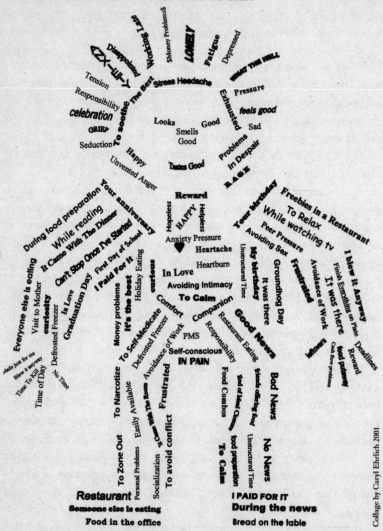

Collage by Caryl Ehrlich 2001

ating new and constructive responses to replace your old and destructive ones. This is called *repatterning*.

I might have missed one of your *Possible Pitfalls*, but you get the idea. Add yours to the above list if it's not here. Observe how you eat when you're up or down, alone or with friends. We even eat differently with men, differently with women, and another way with children. These pitfalls might be because of emotions, circumstances, or just because it's there or you're there, in the neighborhood where your favorite something is prepared as nowhere else in the world! Pitfalls can be any of these things or all of these things.

None of the Pitfalls listed above are hunger. And if it's not hunger, it's not a reason to eat.

What are *your* Possible Pitfalls? Circle your most troublesome:

- _____   • _____
- _____   • _____
- _____   • _____
- _____   • _____
- _____   • _____
- _____   • _____

Setting Your Goal

> *What people say you cannot do, you try and find you*
> *can.* (Henry David Thoreau)

Let's take another stab at the goal you began writing earlier. "I _____ [insert your full name], want to weigh _____ pounds [insert your goal weight. Go for it!], because" and then write every reason, whether it is mental, emotional, spiritual, nutritional, or medical why you want to reach your weight-loss goal.

Why are you reading about weight loss on a beautiful (snowy, rainy) Monday (Tuesday, Wednesday) morning (afternoon, evening), in the middle of May (June, July, December)?

You may not want to set a goal. You may have given the scale power to judge if you are doing things less perfectly than you thought you should. It's just a number. It's a starting point.

Setting an official goal makes it concrete. Then you can take some of the baby steps necessary to move you toward the next steps.

An example might be, "I want to fit easily into all the clothes in my closet, to feel in control, to feel sexier, be happier, look pretty/handsome, more confident. I want to be able to go shopping in any clothing store. I want to feel proud of how I look when I walk into a room. I want to get back into sports, to play with my children, to have more stamina." Embellish on this theme. It helps to write it down. It is the first step in making a real commitment.

Make a commitment to your goal. Make it your *new* ritual. Think it. Say it. Shout it. Enunciate the words clearly. Let me hear it. Walt Disney said, "If you can dream it, you can do it." You can create any outcome you desire. Dream it, *and* do it.

I am not a runner, yet every year, I watch the New York City Marathon covered on local TV, or I listen to all-news radio. I'd hear about Mrs. Koplowitz, a woman with cerebral palsy who 20 or so hours after the start of the race crossed the finish line. It never mattered to her that she didn't win, only that she took the first steps, then another and another until she finished the race. Mrs. Koplowitz inspires me. Against great odds, she never gave up. Do you give up too soon?

Setting a goal in writing helps you create a more successful outcome.

Water, Water, Water

Water, water, everywhere, and you should be drinking a gallon or more of it daily—eight to ten (8-ounce) glasses *in addition* to any coffee, tea, soda, or alcohol you might be drinking. Every time the phone rings, take a sip, and each time the glass is empty, fill it up.

The body needs a gallon or more of water each day to lubricate the joints, irrigate the bowel, act as a coolant, bring nutrition to where it is needed. Water flushes toxins out of the body. It's great for the complexion, and if you perspire during a physical workout, you need water to rehydrate the system. If you're not drinking the requisite eight to ten glasses of water each day, you may be unduly fatigued because dehydration can be a major contributing factor to fatigue. Hands down, water is the best thirst quencher. So if you're hungry, eat. And if you're thirsty, drink water.

You have to see it to use it, so get a pretty water goblet or cup for your home and office. Seeing the same glass or cup every day will trigger your habit to drink the water in it. If you're traveling in a car or going to a movie, take water along in the plastic bottle in which it was purchased, or take a cup you can fill at a water fountain.

Carry a bottle of water on the plane or train. Keep the glass or bottle of water in the same place in your office and your home every day. I keep a bottle by my computer, one near my bed, and one on an end table in my office, near the chair in which I sit. I also keep stacks of plastic cups near the sinks in my bathroom, kitchen, and office. If you drink it, you won't be able to go for very long without wanting it. With each sip of water, think what a healthy thing you're doing for yourself by drinking it rather than all those caffeine-filled, chemical-drenched, sodium-laden other beverages.

Drink water with ice, without ice, or—with a very special nod to my wonderful late grandmother Annie—*hot* (*sans* tea bag or lemon). It's wonderful in wintertime on a cold, snowy morning. And when my hands are cold, I wrap them around a cup of hot water and enjoy the warmth.

> We sit in the library. Lee Radziwill pours me a cup of coffee. . . . It is 4 in the afternoon. Radziwill drinks hot water from a white teacup. (*William Norwich interviews Lee Radziwill,* New York Times Magazine, *Oct. 22, 2000*)

Sometimes when you want something warm, you continue the coffee-drinking ritual, even though hot water might be equally enjoyable, maybe even better. Try not to compare water, whether hot or cold, with coffee or tea. Think of hot water as *another* beverage, different from the others.

As reported in the *New York Times* on January 4, 1998, when the actress Bai Ling was being fitted in the V.I.P. dressing rooms at the Versace atelier, she balanced a red and gold cup and saucer of hot water, which she had asked for when she arrived. The *New York Observer* mentioned that although Donna Karan has the DKNY blend coffee, she doesn't drink coffee; she drinks only hot water.

If you succumb to the addictive qualities of caffeine in coffee or tea (even decaf has caffeine in it, and tea is chock full of caffeine unless it specifically says caffeine free on the label), make sure you try to alter this behavior. If you must drink coffee, pour less each time and leave a swallow or two in the cup. Order water at the time you order any other beverage, and sip first from one glass, then the other until you're almost finished, then switch to water exclusively. It feels good, tastes good, and is one more nice thing you can do for yourself to contribute to your good health.

You might think you won't be able to drink that much water. You're not used to using those bladder and kidney muscles yet. It might take a little time to build your water-drinking habit from four glasses to five, five to six, and six to eight or ten. You might imagine you'll always be running to the bathroom.

Now I feel like a camel. I went from almost no water to eight to ten or more glasses each day. I am comfortable with the amount of water I drink, and I feel uncomfortable when I don't have the amount to which I'm now accustomed.

You use up water throughout the day when you speak, perspire, and urinate. By the time your mouth is dry, you're already running low inside, although you may not be aware of it. For every glass of wine you drink, your body loses double the amount in water, because alcohol makes your kidneys excrete rather than reuse water from the body. And yet water is the only nutrient the body doesn't crave. An atmosphere needs to be created for this to happen.

Larry S. struggled at the beginning with his water consumption, but he stuck with it and eventually he would leave a message on my answering machine with his weekly positive story that began, "Aquaman is calling."

There is water, and *everything else* is food. Therefore, Perrier, Pellegrino (and other brands of non-flat water), club soda, seltzer, and the like are all considered beverages and may be consumed (or not) as part of a meal. You can have water—flat water—as much as you want, all day long.

Water can be found everywhere and is most often free. It is an excellent food-free tool for repatterning; it's something to hold onto during a socially anxious cocktail party—something you can go and get, something you can drink.

Drink one glass upon awakening, one before bedtime, and keep one on your desk during the day and on your night table at night. You should drink a glass or two of water before or during every meal. To keep track of how many glasses of water you've had during the day, you might place ten pennies in one pocket and transfer one to the other pocket as you finish each glass. If there are any leftover pennies at the end of the day, drink the equivalent number of glasses before you retire for the evening.

Use water when you are bored, anxious, and tired, too. It can act as a life raft when the journey is uncomfortable.

At the beginning, I was at dinner with a table full of people and feeling a little nervous about revealing my taste for hot water at the end of the meal. I really didn't want to explain or defend my choice to anyone. When the waiter came for the coffee order, I responded softly by asking for hot water. The weathered waiter, inured to eccentricity by years of waiting tables in New York City, repeated the order without skipping a beat: "Three coffees, two teas, and a hot water. Anything else?" We all shook our heads, no. He walked away, and we continued our conversation.

Create your own new ritual with water. It is wonderful. Drink it!

> Drinking water is not only healthy but easy. The sour
> stomach I used to feel after pouring coffee and diet soda
> into me is no more. On a practical note, I've learned to
> always request an aisle seat on airplanes, anticipating
> the more frequent need to use the lavatory. (*Simon N.*)

> I've become a water freak. At first I hated the idea of
> drinking water—how flat, how bland! But now, if I go
> for an hour without having at least a few sips, my
> mouth feels dry and uncomfortable. It's probably the
> most important thing I do for myself. (*Janice L.*)

I adore the H_2O goddess. She conquers boredom,
impatience, and false hunger and speeds those fat cells
out of my body. It's become almost effortless to keep
the water flowing—a huge adjustment that is an important Quantum Leap [we'll discuss that later].
(*Gladys C.*)

Anticipate and Plan Ahead

"I guess I think I can handle any food situation if I put my mind to it,"
Sally G. sighs. "Then I stop off and buy cookies and ice cream on my
way home from work. My plan is to have only some of it, but once I start
eating, I just can't stop until everything that's not nailed down is gone.

"Plus, I get invited to a lot of food-related functions: dinner at a
friend's, business lunches. My kid's school is always raising money with
a bake sale."

When it comes to losing weight, you have to get out of denial and acknowledge that sometimes certain foods, or restaurants, or even situations and people can trigger overeating. In Sally's case, one of her trigger
events is the trip home from work. She takes the same route past the
same food emporium every day. Her car almost drives itself into the
parking lot of the place where she buys her ice cream and cookies, just as
every morning the car seems to stop off on its own for her bagel and coffee fix. When it comes to trigger situations, you might have a yen for dry
noodles when in a Chinese restaurant because you've been conditioned
to expect them, but you'd never think of dry noodles in a fish restaurant,
because there you'd be swimming upstream toward the clam chowder.

Anticipate where you're going. If you know you drive past the doughnut
place on the way to work every morning, take another route. If you leave
your bus and walk directly to the snack bar on the way to your children's
school, cross the street first, and don't cross back until you need to get
back on the bus.

Think about what is going to be served when you get to where you're
going. The more information you have, the easier it is to make choices
prior to the seductive sights and smells. If you know what you're doing
in advance, you'll be less tempted to compromise your weight-loss goals.

When I suggested to Sally that she call ahead and maybe hint about some food she'd feel comfortable eating, she became agitated: "I could never do that to a friend," she snapped. Yet you've probably asked friends you've invited to dinner about their food preferences, allergies, and the like when you're making dinner for them. Someone who is going to cook for you anyway would prefer to know the truth about what you like rather than have you pretend to enjoy the anchovy soup when you really gag at the thought of it.

Some food is pretty mediocre or downright dreadful, yet you nevertheless end up eating it, and in ridiculous quantity, just because it's free or because someone you like made it just for you or because you didn't give it any thought prior to the encounter.

Is the restaurant known for enormous portion sizes? Does the recipe usually yield leftovers? Are you bringing your favorite dessert to a friend's house for yourself? Are you still eating the horrible airline food? What are *your* automatic habits of thought and action?

On a recent no-frills airline flight from New York to Atlanta, nothing but pretzels was offered one hour into a two and a half hour flight. It was an afternoon trip, so the fact that there was no food was of no concern to me. The return flight, however, left the airport at 8:15 P.M. (9:00 o'clock until we were airborne), and wasn't I happy that my brother and sister-in-law had made a plate of sliced turkey for me, which I'd salted, peppered, and cut into manageable squares for the trip home. Since they didn't have any plastic forks, I chose pretty party toothpicks and happy birthday napkins, which made my dinner more festive. My airplane seatmates looked longingly at my delicious dinner while commenting that they should have done the same thing. The plane landed at 11:30 P.M., and I didn't get back to my apartment until after midnight. Had I not planned in advance, I would have been starving by the time I arrived home. As it was, I wasn't hungry at all.

Plan which foods you're going to have at each meal. Instead of taking everything that is offered, say *no thanks* to some of the more common courses. Your hosts want you to have a good time—*not* be so full you won't be able to function. Saying *no thanks* to a salad or bread or to all but a few bites of something is perfectly acceptable.

At home, keep small cans of tuna, salmon, and sardines in the cabinet— good nutrition in easily accessible, constant-portion sizes. Also have on hand a variety of soups, cereals, and eggs in the fridge. Sliced turkey is versatile too.

When in a restaurant, order à la carte, so you won't feel compelled to eat everything just because it came with the dinner.

There is nothing wrong with asking the waiter to remove a basket of bread. If your companion wants the bread, put it on that side of the table and make a wall of water glasses, flowers, candles, and salt and pepper shakers to make it more difficult for you to reach it easily. If you've planned to eat bread at a particular meal, take your portion and then create the wall.

The abundance of food choices seems to increase to the tenth power when you're out for the evening. If it's a birthday or other celebration or a holiday season, consider arriving late to some of the festivities and leaving early at others. You might want to skip a few get-togethers altogether.

While you are learning new ways of making choices, it might be easier to select places to eat where you know you can find what you want.

> Last minute, on the run, catch-as-catch-can eating
> often leads to unhealthy, counterproductive choices.
> This is not estate planning; rather, it requires only a
> few moments of forethought and anticipation.
> (*Norman S.*)

Put your plan in writing, if possible, so you can work and rework it. If you're serious about changing your habits, it's helpful to know what you're going to do each day. Then you can evaluate and adjust—a bite, a slice a sliver, a sip, and a swallow at a time. You might notice that you're content with one or two items for your breakfast and lunch meals, but all your dinner meals contain four or more items. If fewer items are enough earlier in the day when you're more likely to use the fuel contained therein, then fewer items are going to be enough at dinnertime too.

Larry D. gained 15 pounds. He tended to get so distracted by work that he'd forget to eat and then overeat at the next meal, usually dinner. When I urged him to buy some frozen vegetables and salad ingredients to keep in his home and office, he did. I received a call from his wife the

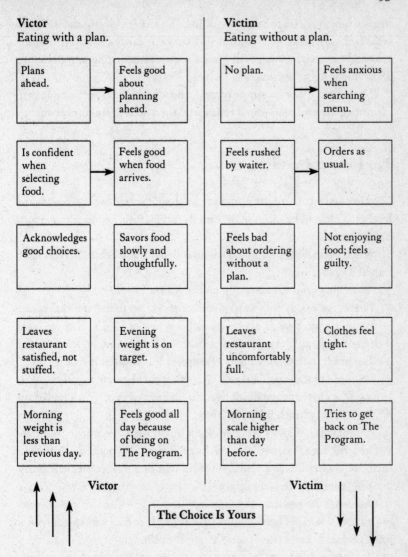

Victor
Eating with a plan.

Victim
Eating without a plan.

Plans ahead.	Feels good about planning ahead.	No plan.	Feels anxious when searching menu.
Is confident when selecting food.	Feels good when food arrives.	Feels rushed by waiter.	Orders as usual.
Acknowledges good choices.	Savors food slowly and thoughtfully.	Feels bad about ordering without a plan.	Not enjoying food; feels guilty.
Leaves restaurant satisfied, not stuffed.	Evening weight is on target.	Leaves restaurant uncomfortably full.	Clothes feel tight.
Morning weight is less than previous day.	Feels good all day because of being on The Program.	Morning scale higher than day before.	Tries to get back on The Program.

Victor   Victim

The Choice Is Yours

other day. She said, "I don't know what you did to Larry, but he's making the most wonderful salads for himself, and he even cooks hot cereal each morning."

The important thing is that if Larry wants to lose weight, he has to think and plan ahead to take care of himself. When he sat around waiting for someone else to take care of him, he either skipped meals or ate whatever was available, even if it was not necessarily the best choice for him and his weight-loss goals. Now Larry is anticipating and planning ahead for weight-loss success.

Think fast. *When* is your next meal, and *what* are you planning to eat?

Anticipate and plan ahead today, and then do it again tomorrow.

No Finger Foods

If you're really convinced that you're hungry, it's time to eat. This means food on a plate to be eaten with utensils (knife, fork, spoon, chopsticks), not fingers.

When I was losing weight, a friend called me at work: "Did you have lunch?" Franklin asked.

"No. I just grabbed a hot dog on the corner," I said.

To me, the words *just, grabbed,* and *on the corner* meant it didn't count because (1) it was *only* a hot dog, a small amount of food, (2) I could hold it in my hands, so it was too insignificant to count, and, (3) it was eaten on the corner with fresh air and sunshine. How could it be bad?

I thought that eating food sold on a street corner wasn't really a meal. It was . . . well, that's the point. It didn't fit any category. So I ended up having a second lunch with my friend.

Another friend and I were walking down First Avenue in Manhattan around 5 P.M. as Paula spied Ray's Pizza. She said, "Let's have a slice." Knowing it was a visual stimulus that had pushed her salivating button, I asked, "Are you hungry?"

"Oh yes," she replied. "I'm *starving.*"

"Okay," I said. "Then let's have a slice of pizza that we can eat with a knife and fork, and order a salad too. It'll be dinner."

"I'm not *that* hungry," she said. What she really wanted was to have a slice of pizza *and* eat dinner too.

How frequently do you eat *Finger Food* and think it didn't somehow count?

When I talk about putting food on a plate and eating it with a knife and fork, I mean committing to the *structure* of a meal.

If you eat slowly and thoughtfully, cutting, spearing, chewing, sipping, and swallowing, you are present at mealtime. You experience the feelings of satiation and enjoyment. The meal registers. Then an hour or two later if you're thinking of eating again because you see or smell something tempting, you know you couldn't possibly be hungry. You just had this terrific breakfast, lunch, or dinner two hours ago. You remember it.

When eating Finger Foods, the reverse happens. Even a few minutes after consuming a Finger Food you think, "I can eat again because I didn't *really* eat. I only had a bagel chip, some black coffee, one rice cake, a low-fat pretzel, and a carrot stick. It was nothing. It doesn't really count toward my daily food consumption because it was so small [or so low in calories, or so insignificant]. It couldn't possibly count."

By rushing through the eating experience, by shoving food into your mouth, by not savoring your food, you fill up your body without satisfying it.

One cracker may contain only 11 calories. That's not the point. The question is: How many crackers are in the box, and how many boxes have you knocked off already and it's only Tuesday in the middle of February, May, September, or whenever?

An apple a day becomes bushels at the end of the year. Do you eat bread so often you could count it in loaves? How much of your food enters your mouth without your seeing it, so you think none of it counts? It all adds up.

How often do you mindlessly put your fingers into a box, bag, or basket of something and put the contents into your mouth without thinking about it? Do you wonder every morning why the scale remains where it was the day before or, more depressingly, goes up?

Are sandwiches, bagels, muffins, and hors d'oeuvres at parties a part of your life? Is a bag of popcorn your appetizer? Are nachos a main course? How many chicken wings make a meal? Hard to count. Hard to know.

Now think: Are you hungry enough to commit to a real meal with food on a plate to be eaten with a knife and fork? Or are you not *that* hungry?

> I finally understand the assignment about food on a
> plate, eating with utensils. Any bite on the run—even

a raw carrot—is totally mindless. I'm not even aware
of what I'm doing. And that goes for all sorts of Finger
Food. Whether it's pretzels and popcorn or canapés, it
just finds its way to my stomach magically. (*Joseph K.*)

I loved these assignments [no Finger Food, use utensils, put food on a plate]. Following them made me feel
like every meal was a special event, even if I was only
eating oatmeal. It broke me of my eating-on-the run,
eating-on-the-street, and eating-in-the-car habits.
(*Karen C.*)

All-or-Nothing Thinking

An overeater is a master of extremes: deprivation or binge, all or nothing, too much or too little, too big or too small, in or out of control. How
many times have I heard, "I can go for hours without eating, but once I
start, I can't stop"?

Compulsive overeaters wonder what is the greatest amount of food
they can eat and not gain weight. They put themselves at risk with all-
you-can-eat restaurants, big portions, and frequent eating encounters.
They end up grossly stuffed, bloated, sometimes nauseous, sick to their
stomachs, and certainly uncomfortable. The frenzy eventually passes,
and the ferocity subsides. They often feel remorse. The next day they go
to the other extreme.

Then they wonder what is the smallest amount they can eat without
feeling deprived and without passing out in the street. So they eat two
peanuts, some 40-calorie bread, celery and carrots, a bite of this, and a
swallow of that. Yet they're still hungry. They filled up their body but
never nourished it. So they want more. And more. And more. They
might feel physically full but remain emotionally and nutritionally
empty. Do you see yourself in either extreme? Both extremes are rituals
of the food addict designed to distract.

We get so busy with the ritual, so great is our preoccupation with doing all the steps in each ritual, we don't have time to feel the feelings that
caused us to seek distraction in the first place.

The 20-Minute Meal

How do you eat a 20-Minute Meal? It's not an easy task in a world full of fast food, faster food, fastest food—followed by quick, instant, easy preparation, package-to-plate-in-3-minutes, stir-over-medium-heat-for-5-minutes, add-hot-water-and-mix, microwavable offerings. How do you slow down in a world full of hurry hurry, rush rush, you'll miss your train, you'll miss your bus? Or you'll miss your kids.

To find out where you are and where you want to be regarding the 20-Minute Meal, use a kitchen timer or your watch to time your meals for about a week.

When I did this, I found my breakfasts were about 2 minutes or non-existent; lunches were 2 to 10 minutes; and dinner lasted anywhere from 2 minutes to 2 hours. Twenty minutes became my goal.

Since this type of eating (slow and easy) was not part of my experience, it took ingenuity and creativity to accomplish it. Often, by the time it was mealtime, I'd be so hungry I wanted to inhale or vacuum everything on my plate. "Slow eating," as I came to think of it, seemed foreign or odd.

First, I set the timer and began eating. I watched the hands on the timer ratchet toward the 20-minute bell, even though I was done in 9 minutes flat. I then made myself wait patiently in my chair until the 20 minutes were up.

I forced myself to put utensils down between little bites, count 20 seconds before allowing myself to pick up the utensil (fork, spoon, chopsticks), and take a deep breath before continuing to eat. During a 20-second rest break, I would take a sip of water before picking up the fork again. Sometimes I needed two or three sips of water to kill enough time between bites. I began to taste food. It wasn't just running through my mouth for a few seconds. It hung around long enough for me to distinguish subtle differences.

Instead of spearing several pieces of food at a time, I tried to eat a little bite of a single item so I could taste the food and feel the texture. Then I'd take a bite from the next category until I'd gone around the plate as the clock continued to tick.

It is unrealistic—not to mention demoralizing—to expect yourself to go from a 4-minute meal to a 20-minute one with a snap of the napkin. Like everything else, it is a process.

My 2-minute or nonexistent breakfasts became eagerly awaited, enjoyable meals. The variety of my food choices enhanced each meal. I was not only slowing down, I was looking forward to eating a meal I'd never before considered important.

Brenda G. challenged me: "I can't make a hard-boiled egg last more than 10 minutes. How do you do it?"

I think it is a good and necessary challenge because anyone can make a large meal last for 20 minutes. It is a skill worth cultivating to make a one-item meal last for 20 minutes. Let's say you are eating alone. Here's how to do it:

- Read a newspaper article, magazine, or book.

- Don't pick up your utensils for 20 seconds between bites.

- Cut smaller bites.

- Finish reading a paragraph (or an article or chapter) before taking the next bite.

- Take several sips of water before picking up the utensils again.

- Read another chapter or paragraph or complete one page.

- Count to 30 seconds before picking up utensils again.

- If you're with other people, ask questions of your companions.

- Wait for the answer before resuming your meal.

- And take little bites, little bites, little bites.

Two minutes became 5, 5 became 10, and finally, about a week after I'd begun putting on the brakes, I set my timer for the 20 minutes, and when the bell sounded, there was enough food left on my plate to mulch a garden. It felt great.

I then practiced making my lunches and dinners last 20 minutes. In a restaurant, I observed the paintings on the wall, the candles and flowers on the table. I listened to the cacophony of other diners conversing. I gorged on ambiance, not food. If I was alone, I practiced eating more slowly. In that way, I'd be completely comfortable eating slowly when I was with others.

A 20-Minute Meal will not be handed to you, but it is a luxury worth attempting. Four or five days can pass during which every meal is relaxing and pleasant. Then my schedule shifts, and I might not be able to eat a leisurely lunch. Dinner is rushed as I need to eat on the way to a meeting. Though life inevitably gets in the way, I try to create as many relaxing 20-Minute Meals as possible.

Breakfast, lunch, and dinner can become an oasis in the middle of your busy schedule. You're entitled to three 20-Minute Meals—1 hour a day—when you're doing something special for yourself. You are worth it.

When I eat slowly, the meal is peaceful, and I often leave food on my plate. I'm filling up sooner because I am smaller. Eating slowly enables me to identify the feeling of satisfaction and to leave something on my plate when appropriate. When I take the time to slow down, I feel stress falling from my shoulders and inches from my waist.

The new way is my comfortable and preferred way. Now, if I eat too rapidly, I feel unsatisfied, cheated, distressed, deprived, out of control, and physically uncomfortable. This reinforces how important it is for me to slow down when I eat.

I used to be the first person at the table to finish everything on my plate. Because I ate so rapidly, I did not give my body time to process the food or send signals of satiation to my brain. It took many weeks of concentrated effort to achieve my slowest-fork-on-the-block status. I am no longer the one looking for second or third helpings, nor do I always look for dessert, coffee, or something else with which to end a meal.

Since the 20-Minute Meal is introduced in the first meeting of The Program, I usually ask program participants in the second meeting what they think of the 20-Minute Meal. One participant, gleefully answered, "Oh. It's so civilized." And so it is.

> I had just started using a fork, and now I'm urged to
> put it down, but I do eat less and it's fine. I'm learning.
> (*Jenny S.*)

> Slowing down was enormously helpful. And writing it
> all down was such an eye opener. Amazing I didn't
> weigh more. (*Olive L.*)

Rules for the 20-Minute Meal

Before Meal

- Stretch before every meal, even one-item meals.
- Say to yourself:
  It's going to be okay.

  I'm fine.

  It will be enough.

  I really want to weigh _____ pounds.
- Deep-breathe once or twice until you're completely relaxed.
- Recommit to your goal.
- Acknowledge that speed-eating does not work.
- Plan in advance the category of food you're going to order out or prepare at home.
- Plan in advance the *Number of Items* you're going to order.
- Plan in advance whether to have a Filler or not.
- Plan the repatterning techniques you're going to use if your original plan is not working.
- When eating, wear tight clothes.
- Buckle your belt on "snug."

During Meal

- Be present at mealtime.
- Cut small bites.
- Eat food individually.
- Don't shovel a spoonful of anything. Take human bites.
- Put utensils down between bites.
- Sip water between bites.
- Ask questions of your companions, and stop eating while they answer.
- If you are alone, count to 20 or 30 before picking up your utensils again.
- Make sure your mouth is empty before inserting more food.
- Chew thoughtfully.
- Taste food.
- Leave food on the plate.
- Ask yourself during the meal if you're still hungry.
- Leave the table if you're eating too much, too late, too fast.

After Meal

- End the meal by putting the utensils down.
- Push the plate one or two inches away from you.
- Push your chair back an inch or two.
- Either remove plate or have someone else remove it for you.
- Acknowledge that what you ate was enough.
- Feel the satisfaction.
- Leave the table.
- Brush your teeth if possible.
- Go for a walk if possible.
- Reward yourself with a food-free present if you achieved your mealtime goals.
- Give thought to the next meal's plan.
- Rewrite this sheet into your logbook and read it during meals when you are alone. If eating with others, read prior to mealtime.

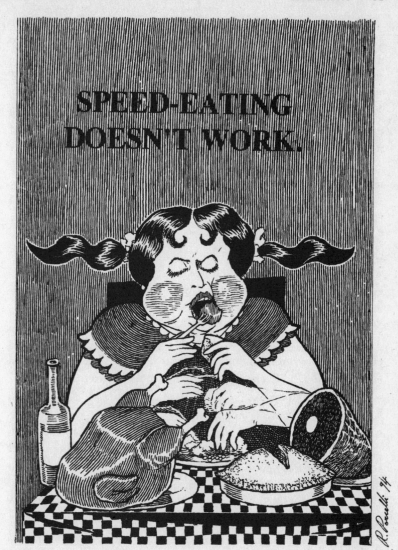

Onward and Downward

"If you want to know where you're going, you have to know where you've been." Nothing could be truer when you are trying to lose weight.

The first assignment I give people who enter The Program is to keep a written log of all food they consume, and to do that they first have to memorize my most important rule:

If it's not water, it's food. Write it down.

In other words, if you swallowed it, you ate it. It all adds up.

And I tell them to weigh themselves twice daily—in the morning upon waking and in the evening before bed—and to write their weight in the logbook too.

Although it sounds simple, keeping a daily food and weight log is my most resisted assignment. At the beginning, people hate to do it.

When I ask people why they want to reach their weight-loss goal, I hear stories of frustration, humiliation, helplessness, and hopelessness. Some people want to feel younger and sexier, others to fit into new clothes hanging in their closet with the price tags still attached. Most want to be more in control and less out of control. Many cry. Almost everyone wants the assignment that will magically transform their bodies from heavy to lighter.

All say, "I'll do anything."

I repeat: "Weigh yourself once in the morning and once in the evening, and write the numbers in your logbook. Then write down everything you eat. Everything. Every french fry from a friend's plate or scrap picked off the table."

"Yes, yes," they say. "I'll do anything."

What I hear the second week is another story: "I got the book but didn't write in it." "I wrote in it for a few days and then stopped." "I started to keep a log but didn't like the paper." "I ordered a scale, but it didn't come." "I weighed myself in the morning but not at night." "The scale registered so high the first time, I never got on again." "I was so out of control with food at a party I couldn't write everything down."

Even the most responsible people are irresponsible when it comes to food. They routinely brush their teeth, pay their bills, groom themselves, and show up at work every day. But when it comes to writing down what they eat, they resist change and become irresponsible. Or their final goal seems so far away that they become overwhelmed by what they have to do to get there, so they do nothing. They choose to remain heavy by choosing to do nothing. They fight change, yet the very act of doing nothing is still an *active* choice—to do nothing.

I point out that there is no change without change. If you always do what you've always done, you'll get what you always got.

They ask: "What do successful weight-loss participants do?"

They do the assignments. When I say, "Keep a log," successful weight-loss participants respond with a detailed food diary.

When I tell them to weigh themselves twice daily, successful weight-loss participants jump at the chance.

It is important to understand that it is totally accepted that changing habits takes time. There is a period of adjustment when quitting smoking. You have to get accustomed to not smoking in all the places and at the times you used to smoke. You realize (and fully accept) that it might take a few weeks, months, or even years to go from the perceived comfort of smoking to feeling good about not smoking.

When learning to use a computer, you accept that eventually you'll get used to all the new terms and symbols. It's virtually a new language. Each bell and whistle eventually becomes comfortable and familiar.

For some reason, you have the patience to wait for success in these other areas, but when it comes to learning a slightly different way of eating—to travel from an out-of-control thought process to a comfortable and relaxed way of thinking and acting around food—you think the result and the comfort zone should be instantaneous, immediate, and final. It is not.

Compulsive overeating is a progressive disease. It took years to perfect all the habits and rituals of your eating habits that have become your addiction. Relearning to eat correctly is progressive too. If you're really serious about reaching your weight-loss goal, get a scale and get on it, and write everything in your logbook—what you eat, what you weigh.

As the scale goes onward and downward, you'll see where you're going, and you'll know exactly how you got there. Then you can do it again, and again, and again until the new way becomes comfortable *and* preferred.

Some participants in The Program initially think it should not be necessary to keep logs, fill out various forms, and review notes daily, but my long experience with thousands of participants has shown that those who do are the ones who succeed in losing weight *and* keeping it off.

Keep a Program Log

When changing habits and rituals, no matter how much you envision the wonderful, successful outcome, there is still *resistance to change*. In other words, you might not be comfortable with the excess weight you are carrying around, but you're comfortable doing the things that keep you where you are. That which you most resist today will seem more possible as you internalize the information by reviewing daily. Since an ideal weight is desired 365 days a year, not just when it is convenient, 365 days of keeping a log is needed as well.

Keeping a log is one of the major learning tools suggested in The Program because it keeps you conscious of what you're eating—not the keeping as much as the analysis thereof. But a log must be kept before it can be analyzed. Because each of us is different, each log is different, and keeping it will help you make a trip from unconsciously unaware to consciously aware. The very act of writing it down reduces food consumption by 10 percent! What a bargain.

I recommend a looseleaf book that is big enough to accommodate all copied information, as well as small enough to carry around comfortably. A popular size is 8½ by 5½ inches. (I use 8½ by 11 inches.) The looseleaf feature enables you the flexibility of organizing materials to suit your personal inclinations and idiosyncrasies. Dividers separating each section are helpful too.

Rewrite related things of interest into your logbook so they'll always be available for your daily review. Feel free to rewrite anything from this book into your logbook, in addition to the pages I've suggested.

Perhaps you can put a photograph of yourself in the book or a picture of an outfit you'd like to wear. Mine was a snakeskin belt that didn't look good on my larger waist.

Write down any proverb, anecdote, word, or phrase that will help make it more comfortable to travel from your present weight to an ideal one. A daily review of information is a gentle reminder, a prompt for what you eventually want to accomplish but have not yet completely incorporated into your automatic way of thinking and acting. A daily review makes the information more user friendly.

A log creates and reinforces a knowledge of which habits are being altered and an awareness of new habits as they are being formed.

A log isolates each day from all the rest. It highlights a moment in the eating exploration of you, and only you.

A log is a veritable road map of hurdles, pitfalls, triggers, at-risk times, as well as successfully traversed foodfests.

A log identifies which reactions to food are really overreactions to something else going on in your life.

A log encourages structure where none was visible before.

A log guides you to repeating the same constructive actions each day until the new way becomes the comfortable way. Repetition of thought and action creates comfortable daily rituals of morning and evening weighing and a detailed record of all food consumed.

The need for such daily written information is increasingly apparent as lost pounds accumulate. As each week unfolds, you'll see what you really did eat. This includes what you do during the holidays, at cocktail parties, meals with coworkers or friends, and restaurant dining. A log reminds you of who you were with and even your level of stress or relaxation with that person or persons. When one woman looked at her log, it reminded her of the week she threw a baby shower for her daughter-in-law and how she entertained a friend visiting from out of town. When my friend Mindy and I meet for lunch, we usually go to a Japanese restaurant equidistant from both of our apartments. When I see that lunch in my log, I remember the visit with Mindy as well as the foods we ate.

As new behavioral alternatives are created to replace the overeating done during many meals, food-related anxiety lessens. If you're thinking about eating but not hungry enough to commit to a meal with food on a plate to be eaten with utensils, you're not hungry enough to eat. But even if you only manage to delay consumption of the first bite or manage to leave more than one spoonful on the plate, write it down. It will remind you that you did it once and you can do it again. One bite of food left on your plate each day is 365 bites of food by the end of the year. That really adds up.

A log reveals frequently chosen items. All these frequency patterns make more sense when observed in the broader context of a week's eating. Do you drink coffee or soda throughout the day, every day? Do you have a cocktail each time you're in a restaurant? Do you eat moderately when out with others only to be out of control with food in your home? In an article about Gloria Steinem written by the Associated Press and appearing in the *New York Daily News,* Steinem said: "Obesity runs in my family; it's our way of coping. . . . I'm a food junkie but I keep it under control. If I had food here [referring to her apartment], it would just overwhelm me."

Frequently consumed foods may not seem harmful, but under scrutiny you might uncover a 1½ gallon consumption of coffee a week, or a 3-quart consumption of wine during a three-day weekend. The cumulative totals will surely startle.

Perhaps the log reveals that all overeating is done at home: "I wouldn't dare let others see me out of control," or "I'm a secret eater." Of course, if you still have a weight problem, your secret eating isn't a secret anymore.

Perhaps your nemesis is popcorn at the movie, but the pattern doesn't emerge for several weeks. "Look at that. I never eat popcorn but went to three movies over the Labor Day weekend and . . ." You get the picture.

You may find all is okay during the day but when finally sitting down to watch television, a path is plowed in the carpet between the couch and the kitchen. The pattern? Watch television, walk to the kitchen, open refrigerator door, eat whatever is there, return to seat with more food, eat it, finish it, watch television, walk to the kitchen, and so on. You get that picture too.

Food combinations become more apparent when keeping a log. Is toast and coffee, hamburger-french fries-and-a-cola, or tuna and tomato your thing? Which items do you choose in combination daily or weekly or every time you eat?

Another habit you might notice is that you're choosing the instant type of food. The pattern of choosing instant packets of cereal rather than purchasing old-fashioned cereals that require a few minutes to prepare is just reinforcement that you're most likely falling into the instant gratification trap. The more quickly you can get the food into edible forms, the more quickly you can put it in your mouth, the more quickly you can alleviate the discomfort caused by a feeling (anxiety, frustration, fatigue) or thought (if I don't eat now, I won't be able to eat until way later)—not necessarily a good weight-loss achievement.

The log helps to identify the times most likely to trip you up. It might not help you with the present trip up, but will help you to evaluate and adjust for the next time. That's the thing with eating. There is *always* a next time.

A log alerts the mind to the Possible Pitfall of a 3:00 P.M. coffee wagon bell and might prompt you to brush your teeth instead as a wonderful and refreshing food-free alternative behavior.

And a log reminds you to reroute around usually encountered stimuli on the way to and from work. I just noticed a new addition to my neighborhood: a coffee wagon on a street corner containing muffins, bagels, and doughnuts easily available to people on their way to work. It's quick (there's that word again), instant, and convenient. How many times each week do you stop off at the local coffee shop or coffee wagon to load up on caffeine, flour, and sugar?

Information found in your log might be a warning signal that sounds a siren: *Alert, alert: Look at what you're doing.* And a log tells how many times it is being done. Multiply the weekly figures times 52 weeks, and the totals are amazing. Loaves of bread, vats of coffee, gallons of soda, bushels of carrots—you'll find it all in your log.

Annie L. gained a few pounds over a holiday and couldn't find anything in her logbook that she considered to be excessive. Balance and variety were on target. However, she annotated her log a half-dozen times in the period of a week that "she'd left food over, left the table when there was still uneaten food, froze more than half the Chinese food take-out, filled up sooner, and constantly had food left on her plate." With all the evidence clearly written in her logbook, it was obvious that Anne was now requiring less food than before. The next logical step would have been to buy less, prepare less, serve less, and eat less so she would weigh less. A good way to think is that she is a smaller person and it doesn't take as much to satisfy her physical hunger anymore. But she did not acknowledge her smaller size or her lesser food requirements until she scrutinized her log. She kept feeding the bigger person she was and remained at the bigger person's weight. If you're leaving food over, the next step is to order and buy and prepare less; you'll eat less.

A log is invaluable in planning a day's eating in advance because what is needed is more obvious when it is written down. If oatmeal is chosen in the morning, it seems as if hunger doesn't arrive until lunchtime, but toast and coffee barely contain enough nutrition to get you to the office before you get hungry again. Team that information with the stimuli of the smell of the coffee or the look of the muffin just sitting there on the counter, and you'll try to convince yourself that you're really hungry again. You're not.

Larry D. told me that his thin wife and two thin daughters were buying a weekend's supply of bagels and muffins for their country getaway, and then they'd leave everything on the counter. Whenever Larry would go to the kitchen to get a drink of water, he'd see the baked goods. He had not created a new response and was unable to leave them untouched.

There was evidence of his bagel or muffin consumption all over his log for several weekends in a row. Once he realized this, we role-played a conversation he could have with his family so they would leave the pastries in the brown bag in which they arrived. He then asked them to put that bag on a shelf in a closed cupboard or in the refrigerator where he was less likely to come across it. In this way, the log helped him become *pro*active, rather than *re*active.

Sometimes you may have to remind the other person(s) of the conversation two or three times. If they still don't change after a few gentle reminders, you may have a secret saboteur on your hands. You may not get the other person to change, but if you're mindful of the tactics, you can stay on your program. The choice is always yours.

A log can also point out the excessive amount of food consumed at the dinner meal. By counting the number of items in each meal, it is obvious that breakfast usually contains only one or two items, and lunch usually contains one or two and occasionally three items. It is eminently clear that the dinner meals contain three or four or more items each day— many times the amount of items breakfast and lunch contain together. This abundant type of eating at dinnertime usually bumps into the next morning, when you wake up and are not hungry for breakfast . . . and the scale hasn't moved (or it's gone up). Breakfast is the most often skipped meal. If you're not hungry for breakfast—and you should be— *you ate too much the night before.* You'll find that information in your log.

Because of conditioning, socialization, and habit, dinnertime is a problem for many people. When making choices, especially for dinner, ask the following questions regarding how you'll utilize the Food/Energy *after* you eat:

- Are you scrubbing the bathroom floor or just watching television?

- Are you on the treadmill or reading?

- Are you wallpapering your living room before going to sleep, or are you just writing a letter to a friend?

A different amount of energy is required during sleeping than during the day when you carry around your full weight. So at dinnertime, you usually need only enough fuel to keep your heart and lungs working while you sleep. The burning of stored fat does that fine. A log indicates when the dinner meal is too abundant. Many eat too much and too late. Do you do either or both? You'll find it in your log.

A log ensures variety, which is not only the spice of life but necessary to satisfy the eye and palate. Texture is another component. Variety and texture do mean different foods, to be sure, but also variety of preparation, food combinations, food choices, seasonings, and methods of serving. Add to your list of frequently chosen restaurants.

Watch preparation. If an egg is fried today, boil it the next time, scramble it a third, and mince mushrooms into an omelette at another meal. Create a wide variety of food choices so there are no particular favorites or usuals, but every meal is different, tasty, and enjoyable. If there are too many favorites and usuals, you'll find them in your log.

Do you see your own eating patterns in any of the above scenarios?

The necessity and helpfulness of keeping a log is more apparent when you identify some of the more abundant meals on your log and think about what adjustments you can make next time.

When participants resist keeping a log, I remind them that what they're doing (not keeping a log) isn't working.

The Food Log

Use a Simple Food Log, such as the one shown here, to record day, date, morning weight, what you ate, and evening weight. It's simple. *If it's not water, it's food.* Write it down. The log does not have to be perfect. Sketch one any size you want, and make multiple photocopies.

Simple Food Log								
Day								
Date								
Morning weight								
What (Breakfast)								
You (Lunch)								
Ate (Dinner)								
Evening weight								

Suggested Meal Plans

Review *Suggested Meal Plans* that follow, and try to make them happen. Here are some things you should know about the Suggested Meal Plan:

- the plan includes a wide variety of foods, such as an All-Vegetable Meal (a meal without protein), a soup meal (thick, hearty, substantive, no bouillon), and an egg meal at lunch and dinner; all these are circled on the Suggested Meal Plan provided. Remember that the reason is so you can tell at a glance whether or not your daily nutrients are in balance.

Variety, taste, and texture satiate.

Volume merely stuffs and bloats.

A Suggested Meal Plan reminds you to get as wide a variety of food (and preparation) as you can. Put mayo in the chicken salad on Monday, and use mustard with your turkey on another day. One day, fry the egg, another time boil it. One day select tuna, another day, salmon.

- The plan includes hot cereal, cold cereal, or egg at breakfast.

  Suggested hot cereals are oatmeal, Wheatena, oat bran, grits, farina, or cream of wheat. (Purchase the kind that needs a few minutes of cooking time, *not* instant packets.)

  Suggested cold cereals are miniature shredded wheat, Grape Nuts Nuggets, or cornflakes. Purchase them without raisins or fruit of any kind; if you desire, add sugar.

- No diet soda or diet product of any kind

- No Sweet'n Low™, Equal™, or similar product.

Why no diet product or diet soda?

When you consume a supposedly low-calorie food or beverage, your *Addict Pea Brain* thinks you can eat gallons of the stuff because it is so, um, low in calories. This type of filling up gives you a false sense of accomplishment. Then when you eat something that is not so low in calories, you expect to feel that same full, bloated, stuffed way.

The body cannot differentiate between real or ersatz sugar, and as many authorities have noted, sugar does not satisfy a craving for sugar; it promotes a craving for more sugar.

- Dessert/fruit, bread, alcohol, and beverages such as coffee, tea, milk, or soda are not included in the Suggested Meal Plan. In advance of any meal, you may choose to have either bread, or beverage, or dessert, or alcohol, *or* you can choose to have none of these.

- *If it's not water, it's food.* Therefore, black coffee, non-flat water, club soda, seltzer, and the like are considered a beverage and may be chosen (or not) in advance of the meal, as part of a meal.

- Drink eight to ten glasses of water each day in addition to all other beverages. Pour a glass upon awakening and another upon arriving at work. Each time the phone rings, take a sip. Each time the glass is empty, fill it. Have a glass of water at each meal, and sip along with any other beverage you may or may not choose.

Suggested Meal Plans are offered to encourage a variety of food, texture, taste, preparation, and satisfaction in order to extract the maximum amounts of vitamins, minerals, overall nutrition, and enjoyment found in foods.

To be certain you get all of your daily requirements—notably calcium—check with your doctor to see whether you should take vitamin and mineral supplements as well.

If you follow the configuration of the Suggested Meal Plans, you'll most likely lose a nice amount of weight this first week. If you follow it partially, you'll still do better than had you not had a plan.

Four Suggested Meal Plans follow. After you've used each one in the order in which they're presented, feel free to use any one of them each week, or write your own. Instructions about how to write a Meal Plan are provided in Session 4.

Definition of an All-Vegetable Meal/a Soup Meal

An All-Vegetable Meal is a meal without protein. If you're eating out, it could be sauteed vegetables such as a Buddhist's Delight in a Chinese restaurant, or maybe a caesar or other type of salad would fit these criteria. In an Italian restaurant you might select pasta primavera or eggplant with mushrooms. When at home, try a baked potato and creamed spinach. I purchase a frozen package of spinach. It's delicious and requires very little effort for something so satisfying.

An All-Vegetable Meal should be seasoned and prepared the way you enjoy it.

Many restaurants create excellent All-Vegetable Meals, showing that non-protein meals can be delicious and enjoyable; the same applies to soups, which should be thick and hearty. Participants say it all:

Soup was definitely one of my favorite learning experiences of The Program. I would never have thought of eating soup for a meal before; in fact, I rarely ate soup at all. Suddenly, I discovered the wonderful world of soup and what it could do for me; it was incredibly satisfying and made me lose weight more than any other food change I made on The Program. I saved lots of money on my food budget as well. You can eat it hot or cold, either homemade or store bought, as part of a meal with a salad, or as an entire meal by itself. The key word here is *easy*. And delicious! (*JoAnne J.*)

It was a revelation to realize that soup was plenty for dinner when I was on my way to play squash. I didn't have time for anything more elaborate and didn't want a lot of food weighing me down. But if it's enough when I'm expending that much energy, why do I need so much food when I'm watching TV? Wow! (*Andy R.*)

The Suggested Meal Plan Charts

Here are some things you'll want to know.

1. The Suggested Meal Plan is a skeleton. Four slightly varied plans are shown here, and also will be repeated elsewhere in the book for easy access.

2. There are strategically placed protein and nonprotein meals in the Suggested Meal Plan. If your schedule compromises the plan, consider switching one entire day with another.

3. Make sure to add salads, vegetables, and starches if needed and appropriate.

Suggested Meal Plan #1

Breakfast	Hot cereal	Egg	Cold cereal	Hot cereal	Cold cereal	Egg	Hot cereal
Lunch	Chicken	Soup	Tuna	Egg	Turkey	All-Vegetable	Chicken or fish
Dinner	Soup	Chicken	All-Vegetable	Swordfish	Soup	Veal	All-Vegetable

Suggested Meal Plan #2

Breakfast	Hot cereal	Egg	Cold cereal	Hot cereal	Cold cereal	Egg	Hot cereal
Lunch	Tuna Potato	Soup	Chicken Coleslaw	Broccoli omelette	Veal Rice	*All-Vegetable*	Turkey Cucumber Corn
Dinner	*All-Vegetable*	Veal Asparagus	*All-Vegetable* Yam	Chicken Creamed spinach Carrots	Soup Side salad	Shrimp Peas	Onions and egg

Suggested Meal Plan #3

Breakfast	Vegetable omelette	Oatmeal	Shredded wheat	Wheatena	Poached egg	Cornflakes	Grits
Lunch	Falafal Cut vegetable salad	Tuna Coleslaw	Chicken Green peas	Sliced egg and tomato	Soup Salad	Veal Potato salad Zucchini	Turkey Cucumber
Dinner	Fish String beans Corn	Avgolemono soup	Soup or *All-Vegetable* Meal or egg	Chicken Brussels sprouts Rice	Salmon Asparagus	Vegetable egg foo yung	Artichoke (garlic butter) Baked potato Creamed spinach

Suggested Meal Plan #4

Breakfast	Hot cereal	Egg	Cold cereal	Hot cereal	Cold cereal	Egg	Hot cereal
Lunch	Chicken	(Soup)	Shrimp	(Egg)	Chicken	(All-Vegetable)	Turkey
Dinner	(All-Vegetable)	Veal	Soup or All-Vegetable or egg	Chicken	(Soup)	Fish	(Egg)

4. Add bread, beverage, dessert, *or* alcohol (one of four or none) to each meal, if needed and appropriate.

5. Remember to Skip and Scatter. This concept will be explained later on.

6. Soup and All-Vegetable Meals are interchangeable.

7. Chicken, fish, and veal are interchangeable. If you don't eat veal, for example, choose a wider variety of preparation for the remaining chicken and fish meals.

People with diabetes may need more than three meals each day. Fourth Meals in Session 2 are a workable solution. *Always check with your doctor.*

Travel with a Scale

If you want to weigh your goal weight 365 days a year, not just when it's convenient, I recommend that you travel with a small lightweight scale. Some are much smaller than the typical laptop computer. It's like packing one less pair of sneakers or shoes.

If you pack the scale first, it will fit. If you pack it last, it won't.

Yes, many fine hotels have a scale in the room, but it's not *your* scale. And by taking the time to take your scale, you are taking your weight-loss program on your trip. It may strike you as a bit compulsive, but in fact, it's an important commitment.

I like the Tanita scale, model number 1623W. The toll-free number of Satisfusion, an authorized dealer of Tanita products, is 1-888-814-9735, and its Web site is http://www.Tanita.com. Also, Rowenta manufactures scales for people weighing up to 350 pounds. For a list of retailers, go to its Web site: http:www.RowentaUSA.com

Not looking is not knowing. Not knowing prevents the feedback necessary to make adjustments and changes. It often means denial. Weighing in twice daily—morning and evenings—is part of my new, thinner, and healthier life. (*Rose S.*)

I had never before weighed myself twice a day, so when I did, it was both scary and revealing. For the first time, I saw the amount of food I was eating. In the beginning, I could gain 3 or 4 pounds a day. Little by little, I was able to decrease the weight I gained during the day, until more often it was the same at night as it was in the morning. I now travel with a scale, something I thought I would never do! (*Errol B.*)

I love the sense of being in control rather than out of control. The daily weighing, writing down food, and making choices all give a structure to my eating. I especially love that I can now go on vacation, log and scale in tow, and come back rested *and* thin. (*Judy R.*)

The difference between traveling with and without a scale is day and night. I feel safe knowing that my scale guardian, my new guardian angel, is somewhere in my baggage and waiting to accompany me to my hotel room. It keeps me in touch with my goals. (*Brent C.*)

Weighing myself daily—especially twice daily—was a great concept. It allowed me to gauge what I had eaten that day, and eventually I knew exactly how much food I could eat in a day in order to lose or even maintain my weight. I now weigh myself twice each day. It's the easiest way to keep myself conscious. (*Loni J.*)

Don't Put Yourself at Risk, Don't Leave Yourself at Risk

Dianne M. and I spoke a few hours before she was leaving on a three-city, two-day business trip. She'd heard about the trip the evening before and was canceling an appointment she had with me later that day.

"Don't forget to pack your scale," I reminded her, "and refuse the mini-bar key, and if it's open, ask the housekeeper to lock it."

"I'm okay," she insisted.

"You're an addict," I reminded.

Any correlation between what you think you'll do and what you'll actually do is purely coincidental. If you're lonely, tired, bored, or angry enough, you will explore the mini-bar. If it is not in the room calling your name, you'll drink some water and fall asleep without remorse.

Of course, if left to your own devices, you never would have purchased the items you think you now must have. You'd never put yourself in this sort of jeopardy, this sort of risk. The hotel employee has put you at risk. *Don't leave yourself at risk.*

Practice when you are without need so you will be prepared when you are in need.

Assignments: Session 1

1. Get a looseleaf logbook—a three-hole binder—and write Food for Thought, Setting a Goal, and Possible Pitfalls in it. Rewrite the rest of these assignments, too, so you can internalize them.

2. Weigh yourself every morning (after voiding) and every evening (before retiring), and enter the weight in your book.

3. Three questions to ask before consuming any food:

    a. Am I hungry or what? (Am I lonely or tired or angry or what?)

    b. Am I hungry enough to put food on a plate and eat it with utensils?

    c. Am I hungry enough to create a relaxing meal lasting 20 minutes or more?

4. *If hungry,* choose to create a relaxing, pleasant meal, lasting 20 minutes or more, with food on a plate to be eaten with utensils (not fingers), and write the details in your logbook.

5. *If not hungry* and thinking of eating, you may be responding to a stimulus. Not eating may cause a bit of discomfort. It also might not cause any discomfort. Many of you may never have tried to "not eat," thinking it might be uncomfortable, but you don't know, do you? The moment will pass whether you eat or not. Taking an action step will help the moment pass more comfortably.

6. Here are some action steps to take instead of eating. Practicing these techniques creates a *new* automatic response to replace your old automatic response.

    a. *Physical*—Move, change location, throw food away, go for a walk, clean a closet, call a friend, go to a movie, brush your teeth, drink a glass of water, walk a dog, cross the street, take a deep breath, read your logbook. Enter here two additional physical activities you can do to help the moment pass (e.g., run an errand, play the piano, knit):

    _____

    _____

    b. *Mental*—Visualize a thinner, more attractive you. Think of the reasons you want to reach your weight-loss goal. Know that eating doesn't change the outcome of anything except your waistline and self-esteem. Envision a relaxed you filling up on the ambiance.

Read and reread your notes and assignments. Enter here two mental repatterning techniques (things you say to yourself) you can use to help distract yourself from food when you know you are not hungry (e.g., I can do it. I'm going to be fine. I really want to weigh _____ pounds).

_____

_____

c. *Relaxing/refreshing*—Take a deep breath; take a stretch break; take a nap, a bubble bath, a hot shower; go to bed early, sleep late; get a massage, a pedicure, a manicure; pamper yourself; go to a museum; read a book; listen to music; sit quietly for 20 minutes; buy a flower; get tickets to a concert; read your log notes; go for a leisurely walk; relax, slow down. Enter here two additional things you can do to relax and unwind to help reduce stress and tension. Such as meditate—stroll in a park—turn off the phone.

_____

_____

d. *Verbal*—When offered unplanned food, say, "No, thank you, I'm not hungry," to yourself and others. You want your Addict Pea Brain to hear, "Oh, she [he] only eats when she's [he's] hungry. For example: I'm fine but you go ahead—So delicious but I couldn't have one more bite.

_____

_____

Use a combination of physical, mental, refreshing, and verbal activities for permanent repatterning. Consistency leads to success, but any action is better than no action. You're trying to create a new, automatic, ritualized response to replace the old.

7. Review your notes, assignments, and log daily. At each note or assignment, ask how you are doing. Is it comfortable? And how you can do it differently the next time to alter the outcome even more? An especially good time for this review is at the start of each day, prior to mealtime, or after dinner and before bedtime.

8. No matter what you thought you should have done, could have done, didn't do, wanted to do, you're only human. *Get back on The Program at the very next meal.* Then think about what to do next time to improve the outcome even more. This is one of the most important assignments. Read this paragraph a second time.

9. Write in your logbook and review daily.

Summary of Beginning Assignments

> *Consider how hard it is to change yourself and you'll understand what little chance you have of trying to change others.* (Jacob M. Braude)

In a PBS special, Dr. Wayne Dyer, author of *Your Erroneous Zones,* talks about not telling others of our aspirations. "The ego gets involved," he says, "then you have to *defend it* and *explain it.*" I totally agree—and frankly, not everyone wants you to succeed either. Secret saboteurs abound.

Don't discuss your weight-loss program with anyone. If they could have helped you earlier, they would have. Unless they have read the words, they will most likely just want to know what foods you can eat. You can eat anything. This program is not a diet. It is the behavior you'll be changing, and that's different for everyone.

In a nutshell, here is the summary:

1. Try to eat only when you're hungry.

2. When not hungry and thinking of food, try to do something else, that is, repattern.

3. Read and reread your notes, even if you think you know what they say.

4. Do the best you can do. There is no right or wrong.

5. Don't get discouraged. Changing habits is a learning experience. You'll get it right a step at a time.

6. Never stop trying.

And here is a summary of the summary:

1. If hungry, eat.

2. If thirsty, drink water.

3. If neither, repattern.

Over the next week, read the notes, assignments, and food log each day. At the end of the week, seven days from the start, read Meeting #1 Review (coming up). Rewrite all assignments beginning on page 77 into your logbook and include them in your daily review.

I Can Do It!

You can do it, and the I Can Do It! sheet shown next will help you believe you can do it. Yes, it may seem unsophisticated. It may seem a little Pollyannaish. It may even seem embarrassing. But you need brainwashing of the positive kind to drown out the negative thinking you practiced in the past.

Say *I can do it!* with a big beginning and a big finish! Nobody is watching you. You want to reach your goal. So read with emphasis and exuberance.

I Can Do It!

I *can* do it!

I *can* weigh _____ pounds. I can do it.

I *choose* to weigh _____ pounds 365 days a year, not just when it's convenient.

I *choose* to feel better and look better physically and mentally about my appearance, about myself.

I *choose* to be free of the excess weight and all the excuses that hampered my success in the past.

I *choose* to succeed.

I *can* succeed.

I *will* succeed.

I *will* weigh _____ pounds and *will* do everything possible to achieve this goal—my goal.

I choose to rewrite my notes.

I choose to review my notes daily or more often.

I *choose* to feel better about myself because I'm worth it! (Read this sentence slowly, three times, because you may have forgotten you are worth it.)

I *can* conceive of this success.

I believe I *can* succeed.

I *choose* to weigh _____ pounds.

I *will* weigh _____ pounds.

I *can* do it!

Rewrite this sheet into your log book and review it daily.

This is the end of the first session's assignments. Keep practicing habits of thought, word, and action. Create a solid foundation, beginning now.

Meal Parameters

Review of Previous Assignments

Date _____

How much did you weigh at Session 1? _____

This morning? _____

Plus / minus _____ pounds?

Was Session 1 information transferred to your logbook?
Yes ___ No ___

If no, when will it be completed? _____. Create
a *Needs Work* page, and write your answer on the first page.

	More Often Than Not	Try to Make It Happen	Seldom or Never Accomplished
1. I keep a detailed log of food.	___	___	___
2. I weigh daily A.M. and P.M.	___	___	___
3. I review assignments daily.	___	___	___
4. I anticipate and plan my food needs in advance.	___	___	___
5. Before eating, I ask, "Am I hungry or what?"	___	___	___
6. If hungry, I put food on a plate and eat it with utensils.	___	___	___

	More Often Than Not	Try to Make It Happen	Seldom or Never Accomplished
7. If hungry, I create a meal lasting 20 minutes or more.	___	___	___
8. When I'm not having protein at lunch or dinner, I choose a soup, All-Vegetable, or egg meal.	___	___	___
9. I choose hot cereal, cold cereal, or egg for breakfast.	___	___	___
10. I choose bread *or* beverage *or* dessert *or* alcohol—one of four or none—per meal.	___	___	___
11. If not hungry and thinking about food, I try to pinpoint the reason.	___	___	___
12. If not hungry and thinking about food, I use physical repatterning to help the moment pass.	___	___	___
13. If not hungry, and thinking about food, I use mental re-patterning; I talk to myself.	___	___	___
14. If not hungry, and thinking about food, I do things to relax and refresh myself.	___	___	___
15. I drink 8 to 10 glasses of plain water each day.	___	___	___
16. I breathe deeply and stretch to relieve tension and stress rather than using food for this purpose.	___	___	___

	More Often Than Not	Try to Make It Happen	Seldom or Never Accomplished
17. I am walking and moving more.	___	___	___
18. No matter how difficult it is to accomplish the assignments, I go back on The Program at the very next meal.	___	___	___
19. I review assignments, notes, goals, and food log once daily.	___	___	___
20. I envision a thinner me and feed a smaller person.	___	___	___
21. I rewrite this review into my logbook for daily review.	___	___	___

If you checked anything in the Seldom or Never Accomplished column, create a Needs Work page and write "Correcting Assignments" on it.

Meal Parameters

To clarify the difference between a meal that is satisfying, relaxing, and nutritious and one that is fast, processed, and less nutritious, I've devised Meal Parameters. They list all categories of food. People often ask me: "You mean I get to eat them all?" I always say, "Yes. But you cannot eat them all at the same meal, and some choices are better than others."

This Meal Parameters is a list of foods from which to choose. It is divided into three categories: a Meal, a No-Meal Meal, and a Fourth Meal.

The foods from the top and bottom of the Meal Parameters list are usually quick and instant, requiring little or no preparation. They are often portable and eaten without utensils. By and large, they are higher in calories and lower in nutrition than the foods from the middle of the list.

These middle-food items generally require some preparation; they are eaten with utensils and are not portable. By and large, these foods are lower in calories and higher in nutrition than those from the top and bottom of the Meal Parameters list.

Here are the Meal Parameters:

Top

1. *Cocktail*—Scotch, rye, bourbon, vodka, gin, or other hard liquor. Because alcohol causes lack of resolve, have one rather than multiple drinks, and always have a glass of water next to the alcohol and sip first from one glass, then from the other.

2. *Bread*—Crackers, rolls, muffins, bagels, breadsticks, pita, croutons, matzo, croissants, crust of quiche or pizza. (These may be eaten as part of a meal, but *no sandwiches*—either open-faced or the traditional closed kind, i.e., bread only on the side.) Use utensils, not fingers. Therefore, if it's an hors d'oeuvre or a canapé, if it sits on a Ritz, it's a sandwich.

Middle

3. *Appetizer*—An appetizer is to be eaten with a knife and fork and not to be confused with hors d'oeuvres; they are Finger Foods. Try two appetizers in lieu of an entrée, or maybe one will do if dinner is later than 8:30–9:00 P.M.

4. *Soup*—Any kind of thick, hearty, substantive soup is fine. Do not use instant packets. A cup or bowl, with or without a salad, is an entire meal.

5. *Salad*—Lettuce, tomato, cucumber, green pepper, coleslaw, celery, sprouts, carrots. Sometimes use herbs, spices, or seasonings. Choose a wide variety of non-diet dressings, including oil and vinegar, russian, french, and blue cheese. Always put them on the side. Dip, don't drown.

6. *Entrée*—Low-end protein is fish, poultry, veal, tofu, and egg. (Low-end protein contains less fat, cholesterol, and sodium than high-end protein.)

Although tofu, a vegetable-based protein, and egg, a smaller portion of protein than chicken, fish, or veal, are proteins, they are not enough protein for the entire day. Think of tofu or egg as a bonus protein. If you choose either one for breakfast, make sure you have a portion of chicken, fish, or veal at lunch or dinner.

Hot and cold cereals do contain a measurable amount of protein but are not considered a protein source. You might occasionally use cereal as a lunch or dinner entrée in lieu of soup.

High-End Protein contains more fat, cholesterol, and sodium than low-end protein. In order from lowest to highest amounts of fat are pork, beef, organ meats, lamb, cold cuts, and cheese. Choose a portion of lean beef once every seven to ten days. It is a good source of protein.

7. *Vegetables*—Dark green and orange, leafy: artichoke, asparagus, broccoli, brussels sprouts, carrots, cauliflower, collard greens, eggplant, kale, kohlrabi, peas, spinach, string beans, squash, zucchini, and others. Choose as part of a meal, such as broccoli on the side, or as an entire All-Vegetable Meal, which is a meal without protein.

8. *Starch*—Beans, corn, rice, pasta, potatoes, yams. Always have with a salad or a vegetable, never alone. (You may have a vegetable without a starch, but you cannot have a starch without a vegetable.)

Bottom

9. *Dessert*—Anything you think of as dessert, such as ice cream, cookies, candy, pie, and cake, are dessert, *plus* all fruit, fruit juice, jam, jelly, syrup, or honey. If it's sweet, it's dessert. Yogurt with fruit is dessert. Also in the dessert category are chips, popcorn, nuts, and seeds. They are quick and instant and have a dessert-like quality to them.

10. *Beverage*—Coffee, tea, milk, or soda but *no diet soda or diet product of any kind.* There is water, and everything else is food. Therefore, black coffee, club soda, seltzer, and the like are all beverages, considered food, and may be eaten only as part of a meal. Flat water may be consumed all day, in unlimited amounts.

11. *Wine/beer*—Because alcohol causes lack of resolve, have one rather than multiple drinks, and always have a glass of water next to the alcohol. Sip first from one glass, then from the other.

Guidelines

1. If you are hungry enough for a Meal, first choose middle items 3–8.

2. Then choose, *or not,* items from either the top or bottom of the Meal Parameters list—bread *or* beverage *or* dessert *or* alcohol—one of four, or none.

3. Foods chosen from the middle items 3–8, if on a plate and eaten with utensils are considered a meal. Note the words *on a plate* and *eaten with utensils.* Food needs to be from the middle *and* on a plate with utensils, or we could end up eating shrimp, rolled turkey, and carrots with our fingers. Utensils and a plate give it a structure and make it a meal.

4. Foods chosen from the top or bottom items, without at least one item from the middle, are considered a *No-Meal Meal.* If you're thinking of eating but you're not hungry enough to commit to a meal with food on a plate to be eaten with a knife and fork, you're not hungry. Do something else instead. No-Meal Meals are about using food inappropriately. That behavior needs change.

5. A *Fourth Meal* of nonprotein choices consists of one smaller item from the middle of the Meal Parameters List, such as a cup of soup, cereal, or a small salad. Protein choices are a hard-boiled egg, ½ can of water-packed tuna, or two slices of turkey consumed at 5:00 or 6:00 P.M. if dinner is to be exceptionally late. Fourth Meals cannot contain foods from the top or bottom of the list. You might find Fourth Meals are helpful between an extremely early lunch and a very late dinner or on occasion between dinner and bedtime if dinner is exceptionally early. Fourth Meals are about nourishing the body. You may have planned chicken, broccoli, and a salad for dinner, but when you work late, have the salad as a Fourth Meal around 5:00 P.M., and the chicken and broccoli later at dinner. Fourth Meals may help those with diabetes.

6. If you swallowed it, you ate it, and it all adds up.

7. First select what you will eat from the middle section of the Meal Parameters list—think of it as your basic black dress or your suit. Then accessorize: choose your earrings/tie (bread or dessert) from the top or bottom of the list.

Rewrite the Meal Parameters and guidelines into your logbook for daily review.

Meal

If you've ascertained that you are hungry, the next step is committing yourself to a meal, with food on a plate that you eat with utensils. A meal should be a 20-minute (or more) affair executed in a relaxed atmosphere (when possible). China, flatware, glassware, conversation, flowers, music, candles, and food are all part of a whole experience. I repeat: *Food is just part of the entire experience, whether you are in your own home or dining out.*

Once you've decided you're hungry, you can eat anything you want, but you cannot eat anything from the top two or bottom three items on the Meal Parameters list without at least one item from the middle. In other words, you must eat at least one item from the middle of the Meal Parameters list before choosing one item from the top two or bottom three items.

The more nutrient-dense foods are found in the middle of the Meal Parameters list (items 3–8), but if you can make these choices with an additional eye toward taste, texture, and preparation, you'll find each meal even more satisfying.

By having food on a plate and eating with utensils, you commit to following a structure. You'll remember the meal.

Why utensils? Why food on a plate? If you eat with utensils, you must look at the food as you spear it, cut it, and move the fork, spoon, or chopsticks to your mouth. You can see the amount of food on a plate. This will give you a consistent visual memory of the amount of food that is satisfying, that is enough.

Food in a bag or box, whether small or big, does not seem to be as much volume when you are eating it a handful at a time, and food in a bag or box is usually Finger Food.

Finger Foods have the seductive quality of not allowing you to see what you are eating. Putting your hand in a box or bag of something, bringing it up the side of your body, and sneaking the food into your mouth from under your chin, away from your line of vision, may convince you that you didn't eat at all. If you don't see it and don't remember eating it, you'll probably forget to log it. But if you do see what you're eating, you'll remember that you ate it and how much of it you ate.

Get all foods (especially yogurt, cottage cheese, and take-out meals such as pizza or Chinese food) out of containers and onto a plate. Use utensils as part of your mealtime structure.

After seeing others look at her with questioning raised eyebrows while she was cutting a breadstick with a fork, the actress playing a thin officer from the planet Vulcan, on the opening episode of the television series *Enterprise,* explained: "Vulcans don't touch food with their hands."

No-Meal Meal

By choosing to eat nothing from the top two or bottom three items of the Meal Parameters list without at least one item from the middle, food combinations such as toast and coffee are eliminated from your repertoire. Toast and coffee is a No-Meal Meal. If you're hungry, really physically hungry, then eating a peach or a piece of toast or a cup of coffee is not going to give you the long-range nutritional energy you need to get yourself to the next meal. Neither is the sugar or caffeine found in a doughnut or soda. They give you only a quick, short burst of energy; you'll eventually crash, you'll still be hungry, and you'll usually opt for yet another piece of toast or a second cup of coffee. Only foods from the middle of the Meal Parameters list will give you the long-range energy you need to satisfy real hunger. In that way, you won't be thinking you're hungry all the time and looking for a ritual fix of something with which to distract yourself.

Catherine N. grabbed half of a grapefruit (a No-Meal Meal of dessert) because she didn't have time to eat a real breakfast according to the guidelines of the Meal Parameters list. By 10:30 A.M., she was sharing a muffin (another No-Meal Meal, this one of bread) with a coworker. She had filled up her stomach with the grapefruit but had not nourished her body in a meaningful way; she was still hungry. The next day when she ate hot cereal for breakfast, she did not get hungry until the appropriate lunchtime.

Lindsey U. was trying to understand the No-Meal Meal concept. When I was reviewing her log, I noticed a dessert she'd eaten an hour *after* dinner. It's a No-Meal Meal because none of the middle foods were chosen at the time she had dessert.

She said she had straightened up the kitchen, checked on her baby, and walked into the living room to eat her dessert while watching television because she didn't have it at the time of the meal. She laughingly considered it a delayed dessert!

No, no, my little buttercup. A delayed dessert *is* a No-Meal Meal by The Program standards. Remember: a meal is food chosen from the middle of the Meal Parameters list, eaten with utensils, of which bread or beverage or dessert or alcohol might (or might not) be a part.

Dessert an hour later? Ask the same question: Are you hungry enough to eat something from the middle of the list in order to have the dessert? No? Then you're not really hungry. You might be tired or bored or even rewarding yourself for getting through an exhausting day. But you couldn't be hungry enough to eat. You just ate an hour ago. If you cannot convince yourself that you're hungry enough to nourish your body again, do something else instead. Call a friend. Get a glass of water. Take a deep breath. Go to sleep early. Read your logbook. Recommit to your ultimate weight-loss goal. Do anything, but do something. You had your chance at dinner to have dessert. An hour later? The kitchen is closed!

What difference does it make if you eat your dessert with dinner or a little later? If you eat your dessert (or bread or coffee or alcohol) as part of a meal, you'll probably take a few bites of the pie, or a wedge or two of apple, or a sip of your drink. But if you eat items from the top or bottom of the Meal Parameters list an hour before your meal (predinner cocktails) or an hour after your meal (a delayed dessert), you've probably digested some of the mealtime lunch or dinner already, and made room for more of the dessert (or more than one cocktail, or a second piece of bread), than if you had consumed any one of them as part of the structured meal.

No-Meal Meals are to be avoided at all cost because you really want to weigh _____ pounds and you'll achieve that only if you eat when you're hungry enough to nourish the body and for no other reason.

Since a No-Meal Meal is an excuse to eat when you're not hungry, examine why you're thinking about eating a No-Meal Meal. Are you bored? Stressed? Running late? What reasons have you given yourself to make this behavior acceptable? Were you thinking of eating because you were lonely? Did the Ring Ding make the phone ring?

Did you think of having a drink after work because you were overworked and underpaid? Did your boss send you home early and give you a raise?

Did you eat the cheese and crackers because someone else was eating them? Did you finish the bag of nachos and the jar of salsa just because it was there?

When Catherine O. was trying to understand a No-Meal Meal, she acquiesced gracefully. "I guess something called Whiz, Ho, Ding, or Doodle is not necessarily designed to nourish the body." She got it.

The No-Meal Meal gives you a false sense of accomplishment. Your diet mentality, or as I call it, your little Addict Pea Brain (and I have one, too), convinces you that *justs* and *onlys* don't count. Your emotions tell you, *I didn't eat anything.* You've convinced yourself the nibbling and picking don't add up. When mealtime comes, even though you might not be hungry, you're absolutely sure it is now okay to eat some *real* food—and you eat again. The danger is that the extra food you've been eating may not show up on the scale tomorrow or even the next day or two, and you may even be convinced you've gotten away with something. But it will eventually show up on the scale, *and on you,* proving once again that you didn't get away with anything.

Alcohol does cause lack of resolve, whether for another drink or more food than your body requires.

Remember the mantra: *There is water, and everything else is food.* If you continue filling yourself with low-calorie and nutritionally low food choices, you merely fill yourself up. It doesn't feel good physically or emotionally. You should be striving to be no longer hungry. If you are really hungry, coffee isn't going to satisfy that hunger. It just adds to your bloat or jagged nerves. Being stuffed, bloated, and feeling edgy is a punishment, not reward.

"But I'm thirsty," you say. "Drink water," I say.

This is a Meal:

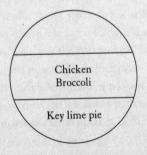

Chicken
Broccoli

Key lime pie

This is a No-Meal Meal. There is no food chosen from the middle:

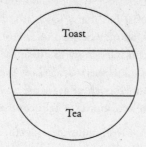

A Fourth Meal

As you learn how far certain foods will take you while you are in a weight-losing mode, you might need nourishment between breakfast and lunch if breakfast was particularly early and lunch was particularly late. Another time you could need additional food might be at 5:00 or 6:00 P.M. if dinner is to be later than planned. For example, you might have had lunch at noon and planned on dinner at 6:30 P.M. Your friends called to say they couldn't meet you until 8:00 p.m. This is a good time to have a Fourth Meal. Fourth Meals are always eaten with utensils, are always only one item from the middle of the Meal Parameters list, and they never contain foods from the top or bottom. Fourth Meals are about nourishing the body. Because food is fuel, the later you eat, the less need you have for fuel and the less chance you have of burning it off before bedtime.

All Fourth Meals should be on a plate and eaten slowly and thoughtfully. All meals should last a minimum of 20 minutes.

Notice that Fourth Meal portion sizes are relatively small to show you that often, even a few bites of something nutritionally dense will (most likely) do the trick.

Fourth Meal foods are always chosen from the middle of the Meal Parameters list. This is important. Don't confuse Fourth Meals with No-Meal Meals. No-Meal Meals occur when foods are chosen exclusively from the top or bottom of the Meal Parameters list. Coffee, crackers, a piece of fruit, or a before-dinner drink fit this category. It's the thought of a No-Meal Meal that you want to repattern out of your head.

If you have diabetes, you might need a Fourth Meal from time to time.

The Meal Parameters list has many foods that have been categorized differently from what you may be used to. It is a good idea to read and memorize the list so you will know the definition of each category of food. Then reread the Guidelines to learn how everything fits into place. Based on the Meal Parameters, there are some ways this weight-loss program differs from more traditional weight control dogma:

- Bread/cereal/potato (often lumped together) are listed separately, each with different rules that come into play. For instance, cereal may be eaten alone; potato needs to be eaten with a salad or a vegetable; bread may be eaten only as part of a meal; and there is a *no sandwich* edict.

  Why no sandwiches?

  If you eat a sandwich, two pieces of bread are bonded to the filling. The Finger Food is picked up as a unit. The entire sandwich will most likely be consumed.

  If both pieces of bread are put on the side and eaten a bite at a time and interspersed with bites from the inside of the sandwich while using utensils, chances are you won't finish both pieces of bread; you probably won't even finish one piece.

- Here, fruit is dessert.

- Potato (and any other starch) may be selected only with a salad or a vegetable, never alone—so no more fettuccine alfredo (pasta and sauce) although pasta primavera (equal parts of pasta and vegetables with alfredo or other sauce) would be right on target. A baked potato and creamed spinach would also respect this guideline.

- Appetizers are eaten on a plate with a knife and fork and should not be confused with hors d'oeuvres, which are Finger Foods. On some occasions, one or two appetizers would be substantial enough to be considered a meal. Perhaps a stuffed artichoke and asparagus vinaigrette would be the perfect choice when an All-Vegetable Meal is needed.

- No diet soda or diet products are allowed.

I discovered No-Meal Meals while I was learning The Program. I also discovered that prior to experiencing The Program, most of my breakfasts and many of my other meals were No-Meal Meals. No wonder I was always hungry and always unable to lose weight! (*Sharon B.*)

A No-Meal Meal was another bizarre concept for me. Wouldn't I die of hunger (or boredom) if I didn't eat between meals? This one was definitely a struggle for me, but once I got through one day with no No-Meal Meals, it became easier and comfortable to do on a regular basis. And it made me look forward to and savor my next meal even more! Now I eat a meal only when I am hungry enough to commit to food on a plate with utensils. (*Danny K.*)

An Overheard Conversation II

I can't wait to hear. You look great. What are you doing?

Well, I'm working with the weight control lady. She's good. She knows I'm a world-class speed eater, so she's forcing me to slow down when I eat.

Slow down? Why do you want to slow down? When we're finished eating lunch, we have to get back to work.

So I don't go into my food trance and forget what I'm doing before it's too late. I have to put my fork down between bites. Chew thoughtfully. Think about the taste of everything.

What are you having?

Probably chicken and some vegetables, but it all looks so good. And you?

This isn't the best place for me to be. Maybe some dumplings. Want to share?

Maybe we could share the main course.

So what does the weight control lady tell you to do?

Well. I have to drink a lot of water—eight to ten glasses a day. My kidneys and bladder are rebelling. I think I'm leaking—that I'll never make it to the next bathroom. I went out with a man the other night, and he thought I had a urinary tract infection. I guess that's better than his thinking I'm fat.

Do you want some tea?

No. If I drink tea, I have to count it as an item.

Tea? Tea has no calories.

If it's not water, it's food. That's something the weight control lady says all the time like a mantra.

Tea?

Yes. Tea.

So how about dumplings, chicken, and vegetables, and we'll share everything.

Sounds like a lot of food, but I don't have to eat it all. She says that too.

And brown rice?

I think that's too much. Not for me. And eating with chopsticks should slow me down too.

Tell me again. Why do you want to slow down?

So satisfaction can register in my brain. So I can feed the smaller person I am. So I'll stop eating when I'm no longer hungry. I'll actually leave food on the plate.

Why do you want to leave something on your plate? It all tastes so good. But you do look thinner.

Thanks. I'm supposed to not want to eat everything served to me because I'm smaller now and don't need as much food as I used to need. I do understand this on an intellectual level, but on an emotional level, I want to finish everything on my plate—and your plate. And what are those people eating over there?

I see what you mean. So are you losing weight?

I am losing weight, and I'm losing inches too. And I don't feel as out of control. Of course, I ate almost an entire package of chocolate cookies last night, but I also managed to throw out the last two before I finished them all. Do you want the last dumpling?

No, thanks. You ate a whole package of cookies?

Yes. But I never threw anything away before, so something good is happening. Do you want the rest of the chicken?

Oh, no thanks. You finish it.

On second thought, if I eat it, I'll have to write it all down, and I have no idea what I just ate. I mean I know what I ate, I'm just not sure how to enter it.

I have to go back to work. But you are *looking great, so you must be doing something right. Do you want any more of this food?*

No, thanks. Just get the check. I'm going to the bathroom. With all the water I drink, if I don't get to the ladies' room now, I'll have to swim back to the office.

Note from Caryl: My telling of this encounter does not change my mind—you should *not* discuss your program's progress with anyone else.

Suggested Meal Plan #2

This Suggested Meal Plan is one of four that appears in more than one place in the book. They reflect a wide variety of foods. Soups, All-Vegetable Meals, and egg meals are planned once a day at either lunch or dinner and are circled on each plan. Do the same circling when you've chosen them for your meal.

Suggested Meal Plan #2

Breakfast	Hot cereal	Egg	Cold cereal	Hot cereal	Cold cereal	Egg	Hot cereal
Lunch	Tuna Potato	(Soup)	Chicken Coleslaw	(Broccoli omelette)	Veal Rice	(All-Vegetable)	Turkey Cucumber Corn
Dinner	(All-Vegetable)	Veal Asparagus	(All-Vegetable Yam)	Chicken Creamed spinach Carrots	(Soup Side salad)	Shrimp Peas	(Onions and egg)

Assignments: Session 2

1. Continue all previous assignments.

2. Memorize Meal Parameters and guidelines. Keep the lists with you, and refer to them if necessary.

3. If hungry, first choose foods from the middle of the Meal Parameters list.

4. When (and if) choosing foods from the top or bottom of the Meal Parameters list, make sure you choose something from the middle first.

5. When (and if) choosing food from the top or bottom of the Meal Parameters list, make sure you didn't have the item already that day.

6. When (and if) choosing food from the top or bottom of the Meal Parameters list (bread or beverage or dessert or alcohol), make sure you didn't have the item at the same meal the day before.

7. Feed the smaller person you want to be and are:

    a. Buy, order, prepare, serve, and eat less food next time; you're *less*.

    b. If there is not enough food for another meal, leave over or throw out leftovers.

    c. If there is enough food for another meal, freeze leftovers.

8. If you are not hungry but are thinking of food, create as many personal repatterning solutions of thought, word, and action as are needed to help the moment of anxiety pass.

9. Celebrate the things you do accomplish rather than beating yourself up for things you did not accomplish.

10. Make sure all your assignments are copied into your logbook so that all the materials pertaining to The Program are in a convenient, easy-to-review format.

11. Review the Suggested Meal Plan, and try to make it happen.

12. Review assignments daily.

13. Rewrite these assignments into your logbook and review daily.

14. Also review daily any other part of this book you find helpful.

Note: Eventually you won't have a large enough block of time to review everything. I recommend you read your goal sheet and the I Can Do It sheet daily. Then read as far as you can comfortably get to; perhaps twenty minutes a day, or *x* number of pages. Put a paper clip at the point you leave off reading.

The next day, read your goal sheet and the I Can Do It sheet, and then continue reading from the point at which you placed the paper clip, again about twenty minutes or *x* pages.

By week's end you'll have reviewed the entire program four to five times, but every day you will have gotten a hit of it.

The Fillers

Review of Previous Assignments

Date _____

Weight at first session _____
This morning _____
Plus / Minus _____ pounds

	More Often Than Not	Try to Make It Happen	Seldom or Never Accomplished
1. I copied all notes into a convenient logbook.	___	___	___
2. I review assignments daily.	___	___	___
3. I weigh daily A.M. and P.M.	___	___	___
4. Before eating, I ask, "Am I hungry, or what?"	___	___	___
5. I always put food on a plate and eat with utensils.	___	___	___
6. When eating, I create a relaxing meal of 20 minutes or more.	___	___	___

	More Often Than Not	Try to Make It Happen	Seldom or Never Accomplished
7. When eating, I choose foods from the middle of the Meal Parameters list before choosing items from the top or bottom of the list.	——	——	——
8. I choose bread *or* beverage *or* dessert *or* alcohol; one of four or none per meal.	——	——	——
9. I drink 8 to 10 glasses of plain water daily.	——	——	——
10. Breakfast contains either hot cereal, cold cereal, or egg.	——	——	——
11. When I'm not having protein at lunch, I choose a soup, All-Vegetable, or egg meal.	——	——	——
12. When I'm not having protein at dinner, I choose a soup, All-Vegetable, or egg meal.	——	——	——
13. I feed a smaller person and buy, order, prepare, serve, and eat less food.	——	——	——
14. My difficult moments are less frequent, shorter in duration, and diminished in quantity of food.	——	——	——
15. If I am not hungry but am thinking of eating, I take as many action steps as necessary to help the moment pass.	——	——	——
16. I will rewrite these two pages into my logbook for daily review.	Yes——		

The Fillers

A *Filler* is a food that fills you up but does not nourish your body. Bread, beverage, dessert, and alcohol (BBDA) are obvious Fillers and fit the criteria.

Less obvious are the *trough de salade,* the cheese melting into a soufflé, the rice that gets lost in the gravy. Those Fillers are most often eaten because they came with the dinner—the salad with your pasta, the rice with your chicken, and the sprinkle of parmesan cheese on your vegetables— and if you eat these unplanned items often enough, they add up and fill you up, but they do not nourish your body as well as other foods would.

They *seem* healthy; the salad and pasta is certainly healthier than the BBDA. You think you can eat more of it, so the portion size increases. The frequency increases.

> A side salad becomes a bowl becomes a trough.

> Salad a few times a week becomes a salad every day.

> A drizzle of salad dressing becomes a drench.

This is a perfect example of progressive behavior.

It is helpful to be aware of the number of times you choose The Fillers. See if any of the following scenarios or foods relate to your eating profile.

Bread is seldom served in basketsful at home but is often a regular part of your dining-out ritual. It might be the garlicky variety of bread served in an Italian restaurant or the saltine crackers that arrive with your soup. There might be bread sticks in a restaurant specializing in steak or a hamburger roll. Bread appears in both open-faced and traditional sandwiches, as well as crackers used as a base for all varieties of cheese.

Don't forget to count the croutons hidden in a caesar salad or the thick cut of french bread drowning in cheese-covered onion soup. Bread also appears in the guise of fish-shaped crackers you eat by the handful. Even a scrambled egg gets served with two pieces of toast.

Personally, I think there's a lot of mediocre bread out there. Turn down the mediocre, the mundane, the commonplace, and the humdrum. Then when something warm and wonderful is presented, it will fit in with your program.

I like to think of processed flour as "prechewed" flour. Your body doesn't have to break it down. Bread, with "prechewed" flour, enters your system and converts to sugar more quickly than, say, a potato. Nachos contain "prechewed" flour, which is then deep fried. Ditto the dry noodles served at the start of a Chinese food meal.

Beverages such as coffee, tea, and soda are often consumed throughout the day as if they were water. They are not. Coffee and tea are also used as an end-of-meal closure. Asian restaurants proffer pots of tea. Many restaurants provide a complimentary second cup of coffee, often called a warm-up or a refill. Modern offices provide free, to all employees, unlimited amounts of coffee, tea, and sometimes soda.

Do you make a potful of coffee in the morning and sip it throughout the day? Or do you consume an inordinate amount of diet soda (ugh)? I'm sure you'll agree that no one ever got thin drinking it.

Although The Program has a *no diet soda* edict, many participants are very addicted to the *behavior* of self-medicating by putting something in their mouths when angry, lonely, tired, bored, or for any number of other reasons. One Filler Chart revealed an amazing dozen cups of coffee every day!

Coffee and soda contain the stimulant caffeine, which may cause mouth hunger later in the day and into the evening; caffeine remains in the system up to 10 hours after it has been consumed. This stimulation can cause you to misidentify a jittery feeling as hunger, even though you're not hungry. If you must drink a beverage other than hot or cold flat water, aim for caffeine-free beverages—herbal tea or milk—always with a meal, of course. If you're thinking of juice as a beverage, remember that all fruit—fruit juice, lemon slice, jam—is dessert, and the juice tosses out the best part: fiber.

It should be noted here that the requisite eight to ten glasses of flat water is *in addition to* all other beverages.

Why is tea a Filler? Because it fills you up but doesn't nourish your body. If you consume too many foods with little or no nutrition, your new smaller stomach won't have room for the nutrition you need and the ten glasses of water you're consuming. Remember that the ten glasses of water are in addition to any other beverage you may drink. And to make it clear, tea is not calorie free, so your body needs to process it. Always worth repeating: *there is water, and everything else is food.*

Dessert is anything sweet, a category that covers a wide variety of items. It can be fruit (apples, bananas, lemon slice, raisins, melons), fruit juice (orange, lemonade, prune, apple, etc.), jam, jelly, syrup, honey, ice cream, sorbet, candy, cake, pie, or hot chocolate. Yogurt with fruit is dessert. Dessert is often an end-of-meal closure, or you might be using it as a reward because you finished everything on your plate, including your veggies.

Enter potato chips, corn chips, nachos, popcorn, nuts and seeds, and the like as a dessert *and* a No-Meal Meal if you've not chosen anything from the middle of the Meal Parameters list to go along with them. If that's the case, work on repatterning the frequency and portion size more purposefully. Eating your lunch or dinner *before* a movie is helpful. When you pass the candy counter, you'll know for sure: you're not hungry.

Alcohol is consumed before, during, and after a meal and often between meals. Martini lunches, bloody mary breakfasts, and predinner cocktails are, for many, part of an unwinding ritual. Because alcohol causes lack of resolve, it may cause you to drink *and* eat more than you'd planned.

You might use any occasion as an excuse to celebrate with alcohol: your birthday, my birthday, anniversary, the first day of summer, spring, winter, fall. Any day will do. Any day at all.

Salad of the lettuce, tomato, and cucumber variety is often included with a dinner entrée in a restaurant. If you want a dark vegetable, you'll have to order à la carte. At home, a salad is so commonplace it appears on the table as regularly as the salt and pepper shakers. Often, it is not a portion of salad but a whole bowlful. Are you having fourteen salads a week— one at every lunch and every dinner? Do you eat carrot sticks while reading in the evening? While preparing food? They are no better than potato chips if you're eating when not hungry.

"It's only carrots," you exclaim. Did you swallow it? Yes? If you swallowed it, you ate it, and it all adds up. Enough mindless carrot eating each evening adds up to bushels at the end of the year *and* an increased notch or two on your belt.

High-End Protein is generally high in fat. Red meats such as pork, beef, organ meats (liver, kidneys), lamb, and cold cuts are chosen less often these days because of publicized health studies. Cheese, however, is as high in fat, cholesterol, and sodium as the greasiest lamb chop, yet you tend not to see it because it melts into the surrounding food.

Feta cheese appears as part of a Greek salad, and parmesan cheese is shaken on pasta and meat, salad, and vegetables. Cheese is often included as an ingredient in a sauce or layered on chicken, veal, or eggplant. It is piled onto a casserole, and because it melts so easily, you may not even think about its being on pizza (count the crust as a bread *and* the cheese as High-End Protein) or in lasagna (count the noodle as a starch *and* the cheese and the meat in the recipe as High-End Proteins) or in quiche (count the cheese plus *crust* as bread, as well as the other ingredients). If there is enough cheese in a dish for you to taste, it's in there, and it counts. Enter as a High-End Protein on your Filler Chart (shown later in this section).

That said, if you insist on cottage cheese for the calcium benefits, use half of a container (about a 4-ounce portion) of the cottage cheese as a protein source. Make a salad by adding cut-up salad-type vegetables. If cottage cheese is used occasionally in lieu of an egg, put a few tablespoons on a flat plate, add a slice of tomato, and you've got a meal.

"Cottage cheese and fruit" is but a remnant of your diet mentality. Separate the food-combo rituals. If on occasion you have cottage cheese for lunch, mix it with vegetables. Team fruit with a different item at a different meal. Fruit is dessert, *part* of a meal.

If you're wondering about yogurt, everything suggested for cottage cheese applies, but if it has a fruit mixed in, enter it as dessert. For a wider variety of food, choose all items only occasionally.

Starch is frequently a part of a restaurant meal—hash brown potatoes with egg, rice with Asian food, and pasta with Italian food specialties. You eat it because it came with the dinner, or you paid for it and want what's coming to you, or you were taught to finish everything on your plate. At home, you probably don't prepare hash browns with your morning egg.

With these items, the question is not only how *much* you eat, although that certainly might contribute to part of your weight problem, but, more important, how *often* you eat each category of food. The Filler Chart will reveal your eating patterns.

Salad, High-End Protein, and starch usually contain more nutrition than the BBDA, but if they are chosen so often each day that they represent a high percentage of your daily food intake, you may want to Skip and Scatter them more thoughtfully. If you're choosing any item so often that it reduces the number of times you eat other food categories, you are cheating yourself of valuable nutrients and enjoyment. Skipping and Scattering helps you interrupt the ritual you've created with certain foods or situations.

When you eat more of one item than another, the eating becomes mindless, unconscious, and automatic. Ultimately, you are not present at mealtime. This could result in your eating too much, too fast, too late. Reaching your weight-loss goal means rethinking the frequency and the portion size of the items you select.

No-Meal Meals are bread, beverage, dessert, or alcohol eaten without something from the middle of the Meal Parameters list. These four items (whether with or without something from the middle) get tallied in their respective places next to bread, beverage, dessert, or alcohol in the column marked "1st 7 Days" on your Filler Chart. If they are eaten by themselves, however, they are *also* counted as a No-Meal Meal.

One woman told me how she'd been eating only when hungry for several weeks and she'd been enjoying her hot or cold cereal or egg breakfasts, and the *Food/Energy* always lasted until lunchtime. One morning she was running extremely late and grabbed melba toast and coffee (a No-Meal Meal) on the way to work. By 10 o'clock she was lightheaded, very hungry, crashing. It is now clear to her that melba toast and coffee do not do the trick anymore. This information would not have been as clear had she been eating so often that she never got hungry. By nourishing her body with whole-grain cereals when hungry, by committing to a 20-Minute Meal for several weeks, it became abundantly clear that melba toast and coffee did not nourish her body. Her program breakfast of hot cereal, cold cereal, or egg did.

A good first step in understanding how your Filler count affects your weight is to tally one week's Fillers on the chart provided. The totals are often surprising.

When filling out the Filler Chart, it's good to begin in the same place: the Breakfast Square of the first day's food. When you enter your breakfast—let's say you had cereal and coffee—put a tick mark (/) to the right of the word *beverage* under the column heading "1st 7 Days." Cereal is not a Filler. No need to count on this chart.

One woman, convinced that bread was her love-handle culprit, was surprised to also see a twelve-salad-a-week pattern. Because unlimited coffee is free and available all day long in her office lunchroom, she kept going back there too. She did this so often she stopped logging it. She lost track of how much and how often. She must have been thinking, *If you don't see what you're doing, there is no need to do anything about it.* This type of denial is part of addiction. Judging yourself negatively for less than perfect performance is part of the addiction too. It serves no purpose. Remain mindful. Write everything down. No judging—it is what it is—no more or less important than anything else.

It was quite sobering for another man to see his alcohol consumption tally up to sixteen drinks in one week when he had considered himself only a social drinker. A few drinks one night and sharing a few bottles of wine at another function do add up.

When I first looked at my Fillers, I discovered that the number one Filler on my hit parade was a whopping twenty-eight(!) desserts—four a day almost to the exclusion of all other foods. It is no wonder I was 50 pounds overweight, bereft of energy, and physically as well as emotionally depressed.

Many of you might find a high bread count, while others of you might realize you haven't had a salad for weeks. When I mentioned the lack of green vegetables and salads I found on the food log of a medical doctor I teach, he sniffed, "Vegetables are for my patients." The Filler Chart is interesting not just for what you eat but for what you *don't* eat.

I'm hoping you'll begin to think, *Instead of another piece of bread, I'll have a vegetable; instead of another cup of coffee, I'll have a cup of hot water; and hold the lemon; I don't want dessert at this meal.*

By counting a week's worth of food, you are creating a baseline profile of your eating. I've marked a range on the chart toward which I'd
like you to strive.

Filler Chart

	1st Seven Days	Seven-Day Range	2nd Seven Days	3rd Seven Days	4th Seven Days	5th Seven Days	6th Seven Days
Date							
Bread		0, 1, 2, 3, or 4					
Salad		3–4					
High-End Protein		1					
Starch		3–4					
Dessert		0, 1, 2, 3, or 4					
Beverage		0, 1, 2, 3, or 4					
Alcohol		0, 1, 2, 3, or 4					
No-Meal Meal		0					
BBDA							

This is a Filler Chart Master to keep your weekly totals. The next
form is a comprehensive food log—a combination of a daily food log and
a Filler Chart. At the end of a seven-day period, move those totals back
here to this Filler Chart. In that way, you can compare your present
numbers with your beginning totals, as well as remind yourself from
whence you came. Sketch this form, and make photocopies from your
sketch. "The measured variable is the one that improves," says Michael
Crichton.

Combined Food Log / Filler Chart

(Use this as a model, but make your own chart larger.)

Day										
Date										
A.M. weight										
Breakfast										
Lunch										
Dinner										
P.M. weight										
No. of items										
The Fillers										Total Fillers
Bread										
Salad										
High-End Protein										
Starch										
Dessert										
Beverage										
Alcohol										
No-Meal Meal										

How to Change Your Conditioned Responses to Fillers

Tally. A good first step is to tally the number of times you consume each category of food in a seven-day period. Enter the totals of each category of food in its appropriate place on the Filler Chart in the first column (for your first seven days). After the next seven-day period, do it again.

Addiction model. You're not only trying to lose weight and to feed the smaller person you are becoming; you are also trying to reverse the progression of the addiction model here. In a progressive addiction, the portion size and frequency of usage keep escalating each time you build a tolerance for a particular food. The amount you need increases, and the usage becomes more frequent. As you begin to lose weight, the portion size of food and frequency of usage diminish in size and number of hits.

Diminish number of times each day. The most frequently chosen items are the BBDA. Some items may tally anywhere from zero to fifteen and even twenty each week or anywhere from one to four times each day. If, for example, you choose any one item four times a day, cut it to three, then to two, then to once a day.

One of four or none. As you strive to follow the BBDA (one of four or none) assignment, much of this will happen naturally.

Mental repatterning. Talking to yourself is helpful as you choose these items less and less often. Think *Instead of another piece of bread, I'll have a vegetable* or, *Instead of another cup of coffee, this time I'll have a cup of hot water.* Remind yourself, hourly if necessary, "I want to weigh _____ pounds," and remember some of the action steps you can take to help you get there. The moments do pass.

Portion size. Get rid of that oversized mug, and pour your coffee into a regular-sized cup. Perhaps you'll feel fine with a few segments of grapefruit, a few bites of coleslaw. As you lose weight and your stomach shrinks, you should be filling up sooner and will require less of everything than you did when you were a bigger person.

Pick one no-coffee day. As item usage diminishes to once a day, the next step might be to pick one no-coffee day and/or one no-bread day and/or, one no-alcohol day and/or, one no-_____ day (fill in *your* most frequently chosen item). Writing your intention into your agenda book (or calendar) will be a reminder of what you're trying to accomplish. If there are many items you choose too often, pick one at a time and practice not having it one day a week before moving on to the next item. For example, Sunday could be a no-coffee day, Wednesday a no-bread day, and so on.

No multiples. Another technique to aim for is no multiples—no second cup of coffee, no second drink, not another piece of bread after the first, and no second or third helpings, even if it is Thanksgiving. In a restaurant, you'd never say to the waiter, "Maurice, is there another chicken leg in the kitchen?"

Skip-a-day. As you lose weight and become smaller, your food requirements will be smaller too. The next level would be to Skip-A-Day. If you had one category of Filler yesterday, don't have it today. And if you have it today, don't have it tomorrow. Skipping days will force you to seek more variety and ultimately lessen the hold some items have on you. Choosing any item three or four times a week works out well for most people, but High-End Protein should be your choice no more than once a week.

If you are sensitive to "prechewed," refined flour most often found in bread and pasta, choosing it once every third or fourth day might work best. Choosing a baked potato, corn, or a yam every other day in lieu of pasta might be a better choice still.

Some days, having a dark vegetable instead of another salad may be exactly what is needed and will help you achieve the Skip-A-Day suggestion.

If you select the same category of food every day, you're eating it 365 days a year, and at the end of the year you'll have eaten loaves of bread, vats of coffee, pounds of chocolate, gallons of soda. By choosing these items every other day, you're having them only 182½ times a year. That shows up as a noticeable loss of weight and inches. Choose an item every third or fourth day, and the results will be obvious that much sooner.

Choosing the same foods all the time cheats you out of valuable nutrients you'd find in a wider variety of food.

Scatter. Shake it all up. If you have coffee at breakfast one morning, select it for lunch or dinner the next time, or not at all. This reduces your reliance on coffee to get you up in the morning. By skipping *and* scattering, you'll get in the mind set of *Sometimes I have it, and sometimes I don't.* This helps prove that the opposite of "I love this food" is not "hate" but rather indifference.

No No-Meal Meals. Eating only when you're hungry enough to commit to a meal, with food on a plate, using utensils, eliminates a lot of eating *when you're not hungry.* You'll get used to it. Or, as Helen M. said after she successfully sat through a movie without eating popcorn, "Nobody died."

Rewrite these suggestions into your logbook for daily review.

When I drank alcohol regularly and frequented a restaurant near my apartment, the bartender actually knew my usual drink. I was embarrassed to know that someone was watching what I was eating and drinking, that my compulsive ritual behavior was noticed by someone else. More embarrassing was that the cashier in a local health and beauty aids shop knew my usual choice of candy.

I remember deciding to have a no-dessert (candy for me) day, and as I stood at the checkout counter, the cashier reached down to my favorite candy. He put the foil-wrapped bar on the counter, and said, "You forgot your candy." I was so embarrassed that I meekly paid for it along with my other purchases and left the store. Your Filler chart might show this type of behavior, but it might also show that you're not having enough salads, starches, or dark vegetables, and those items might need to be increased.

Yes, I ate the candy, but the next time—there's always a next time—I had repatterned enough that I was able to leave the store *sans* unplanned food. I kept reminding myself (mental repatterning), "I'm not hungry, I only eat when I'm hungry, and besides, I want to weigh _____ pounds."

Spiking (and Crashing)

When you consume coffee, alcohol, and dessert—items from the top and bottom of the Meal Parameters list as a No-Meal Meal—there is no other food to help cushion the effect of the drug (caffeine and sugar). The burst of energy *is* immediate. As soon as you reach the high the drug provides, it loses its potency. You crash. You don't go back to the ground floor but to the subbasement.

Once there, you immediately require more of the substance (caffeine, sugar, alcohol, bread, or whatever else it is you use) just to get you back up to the ground floor. If you do this often enough throughout the day, the up and down Spiking causes fatigue.

You also build a tolerance. You require more and more drug to give you the same feeling you had before. That's part of your ritual wall of distraction too. The cycle continues.

When you eat nutrient-dense foods from the middle of the Meal Parameters list, it takes longer for the nutrients to be absorbed into the system for you to feel the energy high, but you stay satiated longer.

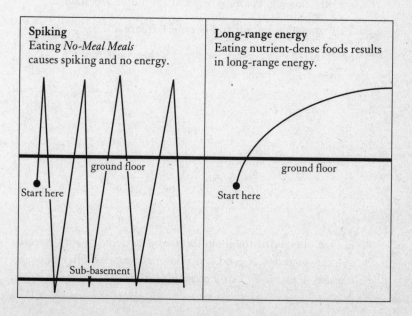

Spiking
Eating *No-Meal Meals* causes spiking and no energy.

Long-range energy
Eating nutrient-dense foods results in long-range energy.

ground floor

ground floor

Start here

Start here

Sub-basement

Most people do not eat a second bowl of cereal, but I often observe others having a second glass of wine, eating a second piece of bread, or drinking a second cup of coffee.

Assignments: Session 3

1. Continue all previous assignments; pay special attention to your Needs Work page. If you don't yet have one, create one.

2. Create a Filler Chart in your logbook, and count the number of times you eat each category of food. Enter totals into the chart.

3. Scatter Fillers from each category, *always at a different meal from the previous day.*

4. Skip a day and scatter foods from the same category. If you had potato salad at lunch one day, skip a day before ordering pasta at a dinner meal.

5. Feed the smaller person you want to be and are:

   a. Buy, order, prepare, serve, and eat a little less food.

   b. If enough is left for another meal, freeze it.

   c. If there is not enough food for another meal, throw it away.

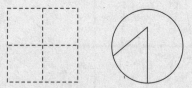

6. Repeat, out loud, throughout the day, as needed: "I want to weigh _____ pounds." A good question to ask yourself after 15 or 20 minutes of eating is, "Am I *still* hungry?"

7. Enter here two difficult times (perhaps evenings, 4 P.M. when kids come home from school, when at a restaurant, weekends) from which you need distraction. _____

_____

8. Enter here the first, second, and third action steps you can take to distract yourself from a difficult moment. Envision yourself taking an action such as breathing deeply, crossing the street, or drinking water, and then do it. _____

_____

9. Complete the Suggested Meal Plan, and *try* to make it happen.

10. Anticipate each day, and plan what you're going to eat, in writing.

11. Review assignments to remind yourself of what you're trying to accomplish.

12. Rewrite these assignments into your log book and review daily.

Suggested Meal Plan #3

Breakfast	Vegetable omelette	Oatmeal	Shredded wheat	Wheatena	Poached egg	Cornflakes	Grits
Lunch	Falafal Cut vegetable salad	Tuna Coleslaw	Chicken Green peas	Sliced egg and tomato	Soup Salad	Veal Potato salad Zucchini	Turkey Cucumber
Dinner	Fish String beans Corn	Avgolemono soup	Soup or *All-Vegetable* Meal or egg	Chicken Brussels sprouts Rice	Salmon Asparagus	Vegetable egg foo yung	Artichoke (garlic butter) Baked potato Creamed spinach

Soup, egg, and All-Vegetable meals are circled.

Number of Items

Review of Previous Assignments

Date _____

How much did you weigh at the first session? _____
This morning? _____ Plus / Minus _____ pounds

	More Often Than Not	Try to Make It Happen	Seldom or Never Accomplished
1. I copied all notes into one convenient logbook.	___	___	___
2. I keep a detailed log of food.	___	___	___
3. I weigh daily A.M. and P.M.	___	___	___
4. I am losing inches.	___	___	___
5. I review assignments and goals daily or more.	___	___	___
6. I anticipate my daily food needs and plan accordingly.	___	___	___
7. Before consuming any food I ask, "Am I hungry, or what?"	___	___	___

	More Often Than Not	Try to Make It Happen	Seldom or Never Accomplished
8. If truly hungry, I create a 20-minute, relaxing meal.	——	——	——
9. If hungry, I put food on a plate and eat with utensils.	——	——	——
10. If hungry, I choose foods from the middle of the Meal Parameters List before choosing items from the top or the bottom.	——	——	——
11. I choose bread *or* beverage *or* dessert *or* alcohol—one of four *or* none.	——	——	——
12. I drink 8 to 10 (or more) glasses of plain water daily.	——	——	——
13. I choose hot cereal, cold cereal, or egg for breakfast.	——	——	——
14. When not having protein at lunch or dinner, I choose a soup, All-Vegetable, or egg meal.	——	——	——
15. I seek a wide variety of foods, vegetables, and preparations.	——	——	——
16. If not hungry, I repattern with an action until the difficult moment passes.	——	——	——
17. No matter what I have done, I go back on The Program at the very next meal.	——	——	——
18. I keep an ongoing tally of Fillers for awareness of my Personal Profile.	——	——	——

	More Often Than Not	Try to Make It Happen	Seldom or Never Accomplished
19. Fillers are scattered every other day, always at a different meal from the previous day.	___	___	___
20. I use a Suggested Meal Plan, and *try* to make it happen.	___	___	___
21. I leave food over regularly.	___	___	___
22. I breathe deeply and stretch to relieve stress, tension, and boredom rather than using food.	___	___	___
23. I buy, order, and prepare less food.	___	___	___
24. I leave, throw out, or freeze leftover food.	___	___	___
25. If not hungry, I take as many action steps as necessary until the uncomfortable moment passes.	___	___	___
26. I incorporate as much physical activity into my life as possible by walking and moving more in general.	___	___	___
27. Every food choice I make reflects my ultimate weight-loss goal.	___	___	___
28. I am feeding a smaller person.	___	___	___
29. My difficult moments are less frequent, shorter in duration, and diminished in volume and ferocity.	___	___	___

30. I will rewrite these pages
     into my logbook for daily
     review.   Yes___

Four Stages of Breaking an Addiction

Nowhere else do the Four Stages of Addiction come into play more powerfully than they do when you resist changing a habit relating to the foods with which you self-medicate. For most of us those foods are the instant, and easily available Fillers: bread, beverage, dessert, or alcohol. For others they are the fatty Filler foods, and plenty of them. You might choose huge portions of steak, hamburger and french fries, or enormous bowls of salad with globs of dressing. Whether it is a basket of bread, a huge salad, or a box of cookies, your body takes so much extra time to slog through the extra food—more food than you're able to burn—that it cannot easily process it. The body wears itself out. You get tired. The extra food enervates you.

Calories are units of energy. After eating your meal you want to feel energized, not enervated.

Eating more than you need causes you to feel as if you are in a drugged state. This altered state zones out the brain and helps you to escape from feelings.

Stage One: Resistance to Change

The Program comes along and says, "Let's not have a beverage at every breakfast. Sometimes choose to have a beverage every two or even three days. Soup is a meal. Put your fork down between bites. Weigh yourself twice a day."

This is scary stuff. You may be thinking you're comfortable this old way, so a new way can't be as comfortable. You erroneously conclude you'll feel uncomfortable. You don't know this will be the outcome—you've never tried the new way before—but you resist change even though you know the old way is not working. One component of addiction is that you continue doing what you're doing even though there are negative consequences.

It is your old Addict Pea Brain resisting change by projecting a negative outcome even though you don't have any knowledge or experience that your projection is valid. The addiction twists your thinking to justify your behavior.

Stage Two: Begrudging Attempts

You join a weight-loss group or purchase a book and decide, however grudgingly, you'll give it a try. "I don't want to do this, but I'll pick one no-coffee day. I don't want to weigh myself twice a day. I don't want to write down everything I eat. I don't want to eat a bowl of cereal for breakfast. I don't want to eat breakfast, but I will because I want to weigh _____ pounds.

Stage Three: Surprise, I Enjoyed It

"I tried hot cereal at breakfast and I enjoyed it. I tasted the most wonderful soup for lunch one day. I didn't think I'd like it, but I did. I had a cup of hot water instead of tea one night, and it was actually very nice."

Stage Four: The New Way Becomes the Comfortable *and* Preferred Way

It's important to know that the attachment you seem to feel for certain foods is not predicated on how much you "love" that particular food. Rather, it indicates how very addicted you are to numbing yourself with that food. Thinking about the food, getting the food, eating the food in a certain way, has become an integral part of your self-medicating ritual. The thought of not "acting out" (not getting your drug) causes you great anxiety. You eat the item (bread, beverage, candy, popcorn, etc.) to relieve the discomfort caused by not eating the item. Consider not drinking coffee and getting a headache and then drinking a cup of coffee to relieve the discomfort (a headache) caused by not drinking the coffee. It's like a puppy chasing its tail.

Knowing there are four stages to breaking an addiction will help you be proactive in traveling through Stages Two and Three and shifting from resistance to change all the way to knowing the new way is the comfortable, preferred way. This information will break you of the food rituals you use to help quell your anger, anxiety, or other uncomfortable feelings or thoughts. Then you can deal with the feelings more directly, more appropriately.

Mini-Review

As each program concept unfolds, habits are being altered by your awareness. Awareness brings choice. Choice brings change.

Asking yourself, *Am I hungry or what?* has opened your mind to the possibility that you're feeling something other than hunger. It might be boredom, anxiety, stress, conflict, anger, or cash flow problems. Painful as they may be, it's not a reason to eat.

As you identify the stimulus to which you respond, its power diminishes. With each click of recognition, your awareness presents new and surprising choices. Friday night family dinners don't seem so problematic once you commit to a plan of action toward weight loss. Ray's inability to leave any morsel of uneaten food has dramatically improved, and she is now able to leave at least one bite of food on her plate. She even managed to go an entire week without choosing second helpings, and she's fine. She's thinking differently. She's thinking.

The Meal Parameters list and Suggested Meal Plans have hopefully coaxed you to create more balance and variety in your eating—to search a menu for delicious alternative choices in areas other than the entreé section.

You accepted the responsibility of keeping a food log, reread the information found in earlier chapters, and chipped away at your previously practiced behaviors of thought, word, and action by repatterning.

You counted your Fillers, acknowledged weight loss by twice-a-day weighing, noticed changes in your body and the way your clothes fit, yet you have not reached your weight-loss goal. It's most likely the number of items in a meal in a day that are standing in the way.

How Many Items in a Meal?

The Program has uncovered the most common reason a person is unable to lose weight: *too many items in each meal.* This might be caused by one or more of the following:

- Inability to acknowledge successful weight loss

- Continuing to feed the bigger person you were

- Holding onto your diet mentality (i.e., it's just lettuce)

- Treating coffee and soda as you would water

- Fear that whatever you're eating won't be enough or satisfying

Study your log. You might see that you're on target with the appropriate number of food items at breakfast and lunch, but that these numbers increase dramatically at dinner. Perhaps Monday through Thursday you choose the right amount of food at each meal, but weekends are filled with many favorite food-related habits, making it nearly impossible to change without a plan. Some of you may realize you're fine at home but are in the habit of wanting much more when dining out—or the reverse is true: you're more reserved in a restaurant, but at home you eat everything that is not nailed down. It depends on which components you use to create your wall of distraction.

Do you give yourself permission to overeat—even plan to overeat by not planning otherwise? Your little Addict Pea Brain will think, *Sometimes you say yes, and sometimes you say no,* and two different habits are created. You're better off being consistent so the more constructive new way of thinking will have a chance to take hold and become a comfortable habit. As the new habit of eating fewer items at each meal becomes familiar and comfortable and *enough,* the old, more destructive overeating habit becomes less automatically mindless.

When your stomach is continually being stretched because you overeat, there is little or no discomfort if you finish everything on your plate. The feeling of being stuffed is misidentified as feeling satisfied. If, however, you continually order a little less, buy a little less, and prepare, serve, and eat a little less at each meal, you'll be a little less. You'll ulti-

mately feel more comfortable. Then, when you overeat, you'll feel uncomfortable. Eventually, you'll realize your stomach's capacity is smaller
than it was; you are smaller than you were, and you cannot eat the way
you did. It just doesn't feel good anymore.

If you're trying to lose weight, it doesn't take a great deal of food to
fill a physical hunger.

Bigger meals equal bigger people
Smaller meals equal smaller people

When choosing the correct number of items for a meal, those for a
smaller person will differ only slightly from those of a bigger person—
maybe just a couple of bites fewer. Don't fall prey to the false media hype
that you can eat unlimited amounts of certain foods and still maintain
your ideal weight. Unlimited amounts of any food—even salad, fruit, or
vegetables—will result in an unlimited body.

How much is *enough?*

It is necessary to realize that food contains units of energy, which
we'll refer to as Food/Energy, and this Food/Energy carries you a specific distance. Imagine a bowl of breakfast cereal and how it sustains you
through your morning routine of showering, shaving, dressing, getting
the children off to school, and getting yourself to work. You're not likely
to be hungry until lunchtime, hours later. Now imagine how much
greater your dinner is, after which you're probably sitting around in
your jammies watching television, reading, at your computer, or otherwise inactive. Before eating dinner, ask yourself how you are planning to
use the Food/Energy contained therein:

Are you going dancing?

Are you plowing the North Forty?

Are you painting and wallpapering your home? My home?

If the answer is no, then you're probably eating more than you're able
to burn before bedtime.

When you wake up, you should be hungry; you haven't eaten for approximately 12 hours. You eat breakfast, which should carry you to
lunch, when you should be hungry. You eat lunch, which should propel
you to dinner, when you should be hungry. You eat dinner. But dinner

need supply only enough energy to take you to bed. You don't need as much food as you do during the day. At bedtime, you need only enough Food/Energy to keep your heart and lungs functioning, a task the burning of your stored fat handles quite efficiently.

Think of your body as a warehouse of stored fat. Instead of eating more than you require each day and increasing your fat inventory, think instead of eating the correct amount of food each day so that you'll burn the stored fat at the end of each day. You want to have a sale of the inventory in your warehouse of fat before you add additional fat on top of the inventory you already have. When your body cannot accommodate the excess fat, your stomach (and skin) stretches.

Having too few items in each meal is as counterproductive as having too many. Aim for a middle ground.

Don't imagine that the amount of food you choose won't be enough. If it isn't, you won't realize it at the moment of consumption; just maybe, instead of getting hungry at 7:00 P.M., you get hungry at 6:45, and maybe not.

If you eat slowly enough during each meal, signals of satiation will occur during the meal. Eat too rapidly, and you'll eat beyond the hunger—beyond what your body actually needs.

The worst that could happen if you don't eat enough at a meal and are hungry later is to eat a Fourth Meal. Learn to identify how much Food/Energy you need for each portion of your day, and if a Fourth Meal may be needed. A Fourth Meal is about nutrition.

Is a Fourth Meal better than too many items at a previous meal? Yes.

If you have too few items one day, don't automatically select more items the next day. That's an example of deprivation in order to binge—something you want to avoid. Your goal is to eat as close to the right amount of food as possible to take you to the next meal or to bed, not beyond it. A consistent number of items will give you a consistent weight. Five or six items each day are better than three or four items one day, only to eat eight to ten the next. Be consistent, and you'll get comfortable with this concept.

When the scale stops moving downward, reduce your choices by one item a day. For instance, if you're losing weight with seven items, stay there. When the scale stops moving, reduce your choices to five or six items daily or a combination of four, five, six, and occasionally seven. And, if five is okay one day, do it again.

To find your daily average number of items, tally the week. Count the number of items you ate each day for seven days, and divide by seven. You will have your daily average number of items—for example,

Monday	7
Tuesday	8
Wednesday	6
Thursday	8
Friday	10
Saturday	12
Sunday	11
Total	62

$62 \div$ by $7 = 8.85$ (almost 9) items per day

Question:

Do you mean black coffee is an item?

How about sautéed broccoli? Is it the same as iced tea?

Is a cup of coffee the same as coffee ice cream?

Is a slice of 40-calorie bread the same as a roll?

If I have pizza, do I count the bread and the cheese as two separate items?

Do tea and crumpets get counted separately?

Yes. Each one of these categories of food is an item, and they are all equal on The Program. When having a bowl of soup (one item) or a side salad (one item), you don't have to count every ingredient. Think instead of a salad portion as a clump of food, a handful on a flat plate. Soup is an average-sized bowl. Don't forget to count the items in your Fourth Meal or No-Meal Meal if you have one of those.

It is not necessary to count the milk in cold cereal, sugar in coffee, mayonnaise in chicken salad, butter on baked potato, the mustard on the sliced turkey. Everything else counts.

What Is Your Magic Number?

Let's assume that at the beginning, seven items per day is your magic number:

Monday	7 items are	0 items over the magic number of 7
Tuesday	8 items are	1 item over the magic number of 7
Wednesday	6 items are	0 items over the magic number of 7
Thursday	8 items are	1 item over the magic number of 7
Friday	10 items are	3 items over the magic number of 7
Saturday	12 items are	5 items over the magic number of 7
Sunday	11 items are	4 items over the magic number of 7
Total	62	14 extra items over what is most likely needed.

In a seven-day sampling, there were fourteen extra items consumed beyond your magic number of seven. If seven is the number of items you need each day (and most people require only five or six items if they're to lose weight), then fourteen items is *two extra days' worth of food*. In other words, you have eaten nine days' worth of food and tried to expend it in seven, an almost impossible task. Even if you are making more healthy food choices, you're eating more items than you need, and your body will convert these extra items to fat and store them.

If your average number of items is seven and you continue to lose weight, stay the course and aim for some sixes and fives. (People who want to weigh 150 pounds will do better with five for six items a day; a 130-pound person might need four or five. Someone weighing 180 pounds or more might need six- and seven-item days. This is not an exact science; there are too many variables. You'll have to figure out how many items you're able to eat and continue to lose weight.

Item counting can become a valuable tool if you tally as you go along. For instance, breakfast is usually one or two items, and lunch is usually one, two, or three. By dinnertime, it requires only simple subtraction to arrive at the number of items (based on how many you want for the day) that will bring you to your planned number of items. But keep it uniform. Be consistent.

How Many Items Should You Have at Each Meal, Each Day?

Breakfast. At breakfast, aim for one-item, occasionally two. A one-item meal is hot cereal, cold cereal, or an egg, chosen from the middle section of the Meal Parameters list. The occasional second item could be the vegetables in an omelette (also chosen from the middle of the Meal Parameters list) or a bread, a beverage, or a dessert, which includes fruit and fruit juice, chosen from the top or bottom of the Meal Parameters list. If you're skipping and scattering your Fillers, there will always be some meals that are Filler free. Occasional is once or twice a week. More than that is frequent.

The Breakfast equation reads: 1 item and *occasionally* 2.

The end of a week's breakfast log might look like this:

	Monday	Tuesday	Wednesday	Thursday	Friday	Saturday	Sunday
Item(s)	1	1	2	1	1	2	1

Lunch. At lunch, aim for one or two items, occasionally three.

A one-item meal could be hot cereal, cold cereal, or an egg, if you didn't have that item for breakfast. A one-item meal might be a bowl of soup, a salad, a can of tuna, or any other protein. The second item might be a salad with the soup or a vegetable with the protein. The occasional third item might be another vegetable, a starch, an additional middle of the Meal Parameters item, or it could occasionally be an item from the top or bottom of the Meal Parameters list such as bread, beverage, dessert, or alcohol.

The lunch equation reads: 1 or 2 items and *occasionally* 3.

The end of a week's lunch log might look like this:

	Monday	Tuesday	Wednesday	Thursday	Friday	Saturday	Sunday
Item(s):	2	3	1	2	1	1	2

Dinner. At dinner, aim for one, two, or three items, and occasionally a fourth item.

A one-item meal might be hot cereal, cold cereal, or an egg if you have not chosen these items for breakfast or lunch that day. Soup is a perfect meal to choose before seeing a movie. Perhaps you're home one evening with a stack of paperwork; a bowl of cereal might be the perfect choice for dinner. I suggest that you try a one-item dinner on occasion and see what happens. You might be surprised.

Two-item dinners might contain a protein and a vegetable, or an All-Vegetable meal might be a baked potato and creamed spinach. I buy frozen spinach, which requires putting a boiling bag in a pot of water and turning on the heat. Two items could also be a bowl of soup and a roll. Sometimes choose the second item from the middle of the Meal Parameters list and occasionally choose from the top or bottom of the list, i.e., the BBDA (Bread, Beverage, Dessert, or Alcohol), one of four, or none.

Three-item dinners might contain a protein, a vegetable, and a starch. Occasionally, the third item could be a BBDA. Vary your choices instead of always choosing one category of food over another.

You might choose a four-item dinner when it's your birthday *and* New Year's Eve on the same day. (My friend Franklin fits into this category.) Keep in mind that the later you eat, the fewer items you should be consuming; if you eat too late, you lose the ability to burn the Food/Energy before bedtime.

The dinner equation reads: 1 or 2 or 3 items and *occasionally* a fourth.

The end of a week's dinner log might look like this:

	Monday	Tuesday	Wednesday	Thursday	Friday	Saturday	Sunday
Item(s)	2	1	2	3	2	3	1

If you're doing your math, you might realize the examples I've used total five, five, five, six, four, six, and four. This adds up to thirty-five items for the week. When divided by seven days in the week, this equals an average of five items each day. I've shown you how possible these goals are for someone wanting to weigh less than 150 pounds. A smaller person might require fewer items; a larger person might be able to burn one additional item *on occasion*. Sometimes it's just a few bites more. George J. was amazed how little he needed even when hiking. But none of these numbers will feel comfortable to you unless you slow down and practice those 20-Minute Meals until they are comfortable.

If, at breakfast, lunch, and dinner, you always have only one item at each meal, it will be unsatisfying physically, mentally, medically, emotionally, and nutritionally. If you continually consume the high-itemed meals (two or more for breakfast, three or more for lunch, and four or more for dinner), the result will be extreme in the other direction. As you move from mindless and unconscious to mindful and conscious, you need to think about the distance food takes you.

A compulsive eater is used to dancing the *I can go all day without eating, but once I start I can't stop* tango. That would be deprivation in order to binge. Aim for a good middle ground of five or six items each day, and occasionally have four or seven.

> This program is the *only* method I have tried that works consistently. The biggest surprise for me was discovering that *one* additional item a day for several days can produce a weight gain. The difference in consumption resulting in gain, maintenance, or loss is not very great. As with many other goals in life, the secret of winning is often in the details. (*Adam N.*)

> Life is full of choices. Choosing one, two, or three items for a meal is one of life's simplest choices. (*Al E.*)

Writing a Meal Plan

The Program consists of a myriad of concepts. Each concept interlocks with all the others in The Program. A Meal Plan is but one concept. These are some things you'll want to know:

- You must have a protein by the end of lunch.

- A protein is poultry (chicken, turkey), fish, or veal.

- Egg is a bonus protein. (It does not yield the same amount of protein as a portion of flesh meat, such as chicken, fish, or veal.)

- An egg is enough protein for a meal but not enough for the entire day. If you have an egg at one meal, make sure to have chicken, fish, or veal at one other meal that day.

- Poultry, fish, and veal are interchangeable.

- Soup, All-Vegetable, and egg meals are interchangeable.

Would you enter a business meeting without an agenda, a plan, a list of things you want to accomplish?

Would you get dressed without knowing the weather, where you were going, or how long and late you were going to stay?

If you enter the wonderful world of food without a Meal Plan, you might get tripped by thoughtful friends and creative food purveyors putting paté in your path.

The Meal Plan is different from any other approach to eating you've experienced previously. Even the writing of a Meal Plan may cause some anxiety because it may seem difficult. It is not. It is different.

Once you work with your completed Meal Plan, you will appreciate its versatility and flexibility. Without a Meal Plan, you might continue to menu-shop in a restaurant or aisle-cruise in a supermarket. Since you may eat any food on this program (though admittedly some choices are better than others), it becomes a matter of when.

If you walk around without a Meal Plan, you do what you used to do. You continue your old behaviors because that is all you know. A Meal Plan is a reminder to at least try the new way.

If you're eating with a group of others, your Meal Plan will help you to suggest where or even if you're going to eat before or after a movie.

Your plan is unique to you. It takes into consideration what you ate at the previous meal, how you're going to utilize the Food/Energy, what time you are planning to eat, and what foods you enjoy more than others. Use this plan if you are eating alone or with friends; lose weight while you date.

Writing it down makes it happen. The plan encourages you to search out a special vegetable or the perfect pear you've planned on eating with lunch. Stating what you want to eat in advance, in writing, helps relieve the food-related anxiety at the time of eating. Knowing that one meal has a soup base will enable you to find it in a shop, have it available in your refrigerator or freezer, or to have the ingredients at home so you can make it yourself. If your plan calls for an All-Vegetable Meal and you're going out to dinner, don't change your plans. There are stir-fried vegetables to be had in a Japanese restaurant, pasta primavera in an Italian one, and Buddhist's delight in a Chinese restaurant. Just today, someone told me of an appetizer of artichokes with garlic and butter and a sautéed portobello mushroom that was one of the most enjoyable meals with or without meat she'd had in a month. These all fit the parameters of an All-Vegetable Meal (a meal without protein). Try to find what you're looking for in a restaurant or the situation in which you find yourself. In other words, stick to your plan.

How to Write a Meal Plan

As you know, there are several samples of a Suggested Meal Plan throughout the book. But for those of you who need to take personal and business schedules into consideration, learning how to write a Meal Plan will prove helpful. Go to a fresh page in your logbook and write *First Attempt*.

Use a pencil with an eraser and draw a grid with seven boxes across and three up and down representing breakfast, lunch, and dinner for one week. At the top of the first column, write tomorrow's day and then continue with the other days at the top of each of the seven boxes. Include the date so you can look back months from now and see how little (or much) you were eating. Remember, this is a bare-bones beginning; then we'll add salads, vegetables, starch, bread, beverages, and desserts to it.

Phase I. Variety is important. Think hot cereal, cold cereal, egg. If you had Wheatena today, have oatmeal the next time. If you fried an egg one day, boil it on another day. Enter three hot cereals, two cold, and two egg breakfasts. I like to set it up so it looks like this:

Breakfast

Hot cereal	Egg	Cold cereal	Hot cereal	Cold cereal	Egg	Hot cereal

Once you've entered breakfast, you're ready to enter lunch.

Where you planned an egg for breakfast, enter a nonprotein meal such as a soup or an All-Vegetable Meal for lunch. In the remaining lunch boxes, enter your protein choices such as shrimp, turkey, or tuna; one of those protein meals might be an egg:

Lunch

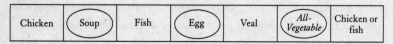

Chicken	Soup	Fish	Egg	Veal	All-Vegetable	Chicken or fish

Circle soup, All-Vegetable, and egg meals at lunch, as above.

> **Remember:** If you don't have a protein for breakfast, it's important that you get it by the end of lunch. By having a protein early in the day, the low-energy feeling that might occur between breakfast and lunch or between lunch and dinner will diminish. You'll notice the difference.
>
> You need a certain amount of protein each day—approximately 5 ounces per 150-pound person. If you eat too much protein, the body will eliminate it (I've heard it called the most expensive urine in the world). If you don't eat enough protein within a 24-hour period, your body will feed off your muscles. The biggest muscle in your body is your heart. Not enough protein can cause muscle weakness, dizziness, spaciness, and general fatigue. This is dangerous. Make sure you're getting enough protein daily. You're better off having a little too much than not enough.

Where you had an egg at breakfast or lunch, there is enough protein to get you through lunch, but not enough for the entire day. Have additional protein at that day's dinner meal. Enter chicken, fish, or veal on the days where the only protein you had at breakfast or lunch was an egg.

In the remaining dinner boxes, enter one or two soup meals, one or two All-Vegetable, or an egg meal:

Dinner

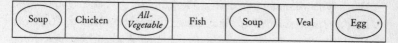

| (Soup) | Chicken | (All-Vegetable) | Fish | (Soup) | Veal | (Egg) |

Circle Soup, All-Vegetable, and egg meals at dinner.

You've completed phase I of the basic Meal Plan. It is a beginning, the first layer. You should have at least one circled meal at either lunch or dinner for each of seven days.

Phase II. Go back over each lunch and dinner meal and add vegetables, salads, or starch if needed and appropriate (i.e., if you didn't have the item earlier in the day or the day before). Add coleslaw to one lunch, baked potato to a dinner, a broccoli sauté here, and an acorn squash over there. Make the meal come to life in the plan. In that way, you will be able to purchase the foods necessary to achieve your plan. If a bowl of soup looks okay the way you've written it and you decide you can do without a salad because you'll be rushing to a lecture, move on to the next meal square. Do this until you're satisfied with your plan, but it's not etched in stone.

Phase III. Choose items from the top or bottom of the Meal Parameters List (bread, beverage, dessert, or alcohol), if needed and appropriate. In other words, if you didn't have bread earlier today or yesterday and you're planning to have it later today, write it in your plan. Using a pencil with an eraser helps you select exactly the foods you'll want for each meal. If I know I'm going to a wedding and plan to have a piece of wedding cake, I won't have fruit with my cereal that morning.

Phase IV. Count the number of items for breakfast, lunch, and dinner. Check the totals with your magic number, and use your eraser to adjust, if need be.

When your plan is completed to your satisfaction, a helpful step might be to enter it into your daily calendar or agenda book. It is one additional reminder of your plan. When a friend wants to have dinner, you can glance at your plan before you decide where to eat.

Work with your suggested Meal Plan, and *try* to make it happen.

It is not necessary that your entire first plan succeed. If you've planned a protein meal of chicken and none is available, have some other protein. The same is true of soup and All-Vegetable Meals. They are interchangeable too. If you plan on protein and end up with soup or vice versa, it will only throw off your protein consumption for the day.

If you ever feel lightheaded and hungry between meals and need a Fourth Meal, choose protein. A hard-boiled egg, half a can of tuna, or two slices of turkey fit these guidelines. It is usually what you need if you feel lightheaded. If you are merely hungry, a cup of cereal or soup or a small salad are good choices for a Fourth Meal.

Almost every food has some protein in it. What I am talking about is an actual protein source. I want you to think of flesh meats such as chicken, fish, veal, and an occasional steak or hamburger as a protein meal.

As you write and use your Meal Plan, you will be able to take into consideration the night you eat late because you work late, the first-of-the-month business lunch, or the demand-performance Christmas party you must attend.

The first week's Meal Plan may fall apart, and you may not feel you want to make or follow a second plan. If you do try to follow it, you will learn enough to make a more realistic plan the second week. The more you use the plan, the more you will realize how helpful it is. A Meal Plan not only guides you to a healthier way of eating, but helps identify items you've woven into your eating life. Are you planning certain foods too often, or are there foods you're not having often enough?

It takes time to build a constructive habit and to break a destructive one. Repetition helps to polish and perfect this new way of thinking and eating and to leave the old way of doing things in the closet with the double-digit-sized pair of slacks. (Eventually, you'll get rid of those too.)

Some Action Steps to Take

When awakening in the morning, just as you look at your to-do list to remind you of your appointments and errands, it is a good idea to look at your Meal Plan.

Plan and envision the breakfast, lunch, and dinner you're trying to achieve that day. Imagine yourself eating what you planned. It is when you do not have a plan that you eat whatever comes your way—whatever smells good or looks good or happens to be there at the time.

When in a restaurant, try to select the meal you've planned from whatever is available. It might take a little creativity on your part—perhaps the garlic spinach with the pasta and salad would fit the criteria for an All-Vegetable Meal—but it is well worth the effort. In creating new habits, the old ones lose their potency. The more you seek out a nutrient-dense variety of food on a menu or at home, the less often you'll want to grab the instant variety of food you've been eating. After a while, it won't satisfy you anymore.

Prepare shopping lists for food from the Meal Plan you've created, and buy only what is on the list. If you are eating most meals in a restaurant, prepare menu choices from your plan and order what you've planned. Which one, two, or three items had you planned on having? Find them. It's easy to get waylaid by someone else's penmanship or ability to write descriptive phrases about tunafish. Before you decide to eat, remind yourself that you want to weigh _____ pounds.

Get the tools. Get the foods into the house.

Buy hot cereals: oatmeal, Wheatena, Cream of Wheat, farina, and grits—the kind *that need a few minutes of cooking;* no instant packets. Or buy cold cereal: miniature shredded wheat, cornflakes, Grape Nuts Nuggets, etc., cereals that are all excellent sources of fiber and are low in sodium and sugar. Purchase cereals without raisins or fruits. If you want fruit (dessert), add it to your cereal on occasion. Eat breakfast in a coffee shop? Most have at least one hot cereal available each day, even in summer.

Try vegetables you haven't eaten in a while. Incorporate them into your variety of choices. When was the last time you had an artichoke? Eggplant? Collard greens?

Include vitamin-rich foods in your eating day. A vitamin C tablet gives you vitamin C. Broccoli contains a large amount of vitamin C plus other trace minerals, plus fiber, not to mention the chewing/crunching/flavor factor. Yumm. That said, check with your doctor to see if he or she wants you to take a multivitamin/mineral and/or calcium, too.

By including grains at breakfast, All-Vegetable Meals, eight to ten glasses of water each day, elimination of waste material from your body should be the most efficient it has ever been. If you tend to be constipated, see if you're eating products like cheese, milk, ice cream, or rice too often; they might bind.

Eat foods high in water, such as spinach, zucchini, cantaloupe, lettuce, squash, eggplant, mushrooms, and cucumber in addition to your ten glasses of water each day.

Take your Meal Plan *seriously.* If you get sidetracked because of the smell or sight or sound of something, work on mental repatternings—things you say to yourself.

Repattern by sticking to your plan. Annotate how enjoyable your food is now that you're not racing through every meal. If you're feeling a bit of anxiety, leave the table and do some deep breathing to calm down.

If at the end of the week you are able to achieve more than half your plan, you're doing well, and will certainly do better weight-wise than had you not had a plan. After a few weeks, you'll accomplish almost every one of the twenty-one meals you've planned.

Keep Program food in the office as well as at home. Have some cans of tuna, salmon, and soup and plastic bags of cold cereal in the cupboard in case you have to work late and you're not in the mood to go halvsies on the pizza with the rest of the crew. Keep pretty paper plates and utensils there too. Then, if the answer to "Am I hungry?" is *yes,* you know you don't have to find a take-out menu or meet the minimum order when you really only wanted soup.

Essentials of How to Write a Meal Plan

- On the days you have an egg at breakfast, have a soup or an All-Vegetable lunch.

- On the days you have cereal for breakfast, you should have a protein lunch (chicken, fish, veal, egg).

- On the days where you had an egg at either breakfast or lunch, you've had enough protein to get you through lunch, but not enough for the day. Those days, the dinner meal should be an additional source of protein, such as chicken, fish, or veal.

- Where you've had a protein such as chicken, fish, or veal at lunch, the dinner meal should be a soup, All-Vegetable, or egg meal.

Summary of How to Write a Meal Plan

1. Use a pencil with an eraser.

2. Make a grid with twenty-one boxes (seven across and three down).

3. Enter breakfast—three hot cereal, two cold cereal, and two egg meals.

4. Where egg is breakfast, enter soup at one lunch and an All-Vegetable Meal at the other.

5. At the remaining five lunches, enter an egg at one meal and other low-end protein items such as shrimp, turkey, and tuna in the remaining lunch boxes.

6. When you had an egg at breakfast or lunch, enter a protein such as chicken, fish, or veal in the dinner boxes.

7. In the remaining four dinners, enter two All-Vegetable Meals, one soup meal, and one egg meal.

8. At lunch and dinner, circle All-Vegetable Meal, soup, and egg meals. You should have at least one circle each day for seven days.

9. Scan the meal plan at lunch and dinner to add vegetables, salads, and starch, if needed and appropriate.

10. Choose bread *or* beverage *or* dessert *or* alcohol from the top or bottom of the Meal Parameters in advance of mealtime, if necessary and appropriate.

11. When the plan is completed, count the number of items to see if any meal or day needs eraser action.

12. Enter the suggested foods into your daily calendar or agenda book. It is one additional reminder of an action step you can take that takes you closer to your weight-loss goal.

13. Work with the Suggested Meal Plan, and *try* to make it happen.

Assignments: Session 4

1. Continue all previous assignments.

2. Keep a count of all Fillers you choose frequently. If you consume them several times each day, diminish to just once each day, always at a different meal than the previous day.

3. If you now consume a Filler once each day, diminish to every other day, always at a different meal than the previous day.

4. Choose one item for breakfast; occasionally choose two items.

5. Choose one or two items for lunch; occasionally choose three items.

6. Choose one or two or three items for dinner; occasionally choose a fourth item.

7. Aim for five to six items or fewer each day. Be uniform, i.e., have five to six items daily—rather than confining yourself to five items on weekdays, only to have ten to twelve at evenings and weekends.

8. Make a point of taking a relaxation break that includes long, satisfying deep breathing and stretching at least once an hour, on the hour.

9. Try to have an All-Vegetable Lunch by Wednesday and a soup meal by Friday. Write your intentions in your calendar on an appropriate page.

10. Copy this session's assignments on this page into your logbook. If you have not done this with all previous information, set a goal to do so.

a. Pick the most appropriate time. _____ A.M.
    _____ P.M.

b. Pick the most appropriate day. _____.

c. Pick a specific date this week. _____.

d. Write statement of intention: I, _____,
    will enter my Program notes into my logbook at
    (time) _____, (day) _____, (date) _____.

11. Review notes and progress daily.

Suggested Meal Plan #4

Breakfast	Hot cereal	Egg	Cold cereal	Hot cereal	Cold cereal	Egg	Hot cereal
Lunch	Chicken	Soup	Shrimp	Egg	Chicken	*All-Vegetable*	Turkey
Dinner	*All-Vegetable*	Veal	Soup or *All-Vegetable* or egg	Chicken	Soup	Fish	Egg

Session 5

Portion Size

Review of Previous Assignments

Date _____

How much did you weigh at the first session? _____
This morning? _____ Plus/Minus _____ pounds

	More Often Than Not	Try to Make It Happen	Seldom or Never Accomplished
1. I copied all notes into one convenient logbook.	___	___	___
2. I keep a detailed log of food.	___	___	___
3. I weigh daily A.M. and P.M.	___	___	___
4. I review assignments and goals daily or more.	___	___	___
5. I anticipate my day and plan my food in advance, in writing.	___	___	___
6. Before consuming any food I ask, Am I hungry, or what?	___	___	___
7. If I'm hungry, I create a 20-minute, relaxing meal.	___	___	___

	More Often Than Not	Try to Make It Happen	Seldom or Never Accomplished
8. I put food on a plate and eat with utensils.	——	——	——
9. I choose bread *or* beverage *or* dessert *or* alcohol—one of four or none.	——	——	——
10. I choose foods from the middle of the Meal Parameters list before choosing items from the top or bottom.	——	——	——
11. I drink 8 to 10 (or more) glasses of plain water daily.	——	——	——
12. I choose hot cereal, cold cereal, or an egg for breakfast.	——	——	——
13. I choose an All-Vegetable Meal, a soup meal, or an egg meal at least once a day at lunch or dinner.	——	——	——
14. I seek a wide variety of foods, vegetables, and preparations.	——	——	——
15. If I am not hungry but thinking of food, I create an action until the difficult moment passes.	——	——	——
16. My uncomfortable moments are less frequent, shorter in duration, and diminished in volume and ferocity.	——	——	——
17. No matter what I have done, I go back on The Program at the very next meal.	——	——	——

	More Often Than Not	Try to Make It Happen	Seldom or Never Accomplished
18. I keep a daily tally of my Fillers.	___	___	___
19. Fillers are scattered every other day, always at a different meal from the previous day and are decreasing in frequency.	___	___	___
20. I consume five or six items daily (with an occasional four-item or seven-item day), with one, two, three, or four at dinner; one, two, or three at lunch; and one or two at breakfast.	___	___	___
21. I often leave food on my plate when it is appropriate.	___	___	___
22. I breathe deeply and stretch to relieve tension, stress, and boredom rather than using food.	___	___	___
23. I buy, order, and prepare less food.	___	___	___
24. I leave, throw out, or freeze leftover food.	___	___	___
25. I incorporate as much physical activity into my life as possible by walking and moving more in general.	___	___	___
26. Every food choice I make reflects my ultimate weight-loss goal.	___	___	___
27. I'm feeding a smaller person.	___	___	___

28. I will rewrite Session 5 Review
into my logbook for
daily review.   Yes___

29. List the three most important things you'd like to concentrate on
this week, and enter them in your logbook on Needs Work page.

_____

_____

_____

Portion Size: The Problems

Portions come in every imaginable size from minuscule to gargantuan
and everything in between. It's plain and simple: if you weigh more than
you want to, you are eating more than you need. It is time to look seriously at portion size.

Just as a one-size-fits-all article of clothing does not fit everyone, a
one-size-fits-all portion of food is too much or too little for some of you.

You are prey to portion sizes of your own, as well as those of the
butcher, the baker, and the chef in the restaurant. Add to that the protein
sizes in your friends' recipes and those in nature's house: fruits (grapes to
watermelons), vegetables (brussels sprouts to cabbage), chickens (wing to
breast), and eggs (small to jumbo). A cut of beef in a supermarket might
be two, three, or more times more than you actually need. If you want
only one slice of bread, you may have to buy an entire loaf to get it.

There are different size glasses, dishes, and canned goods, serving
containers, bottles of wine, and bottles of beer on the wall. There are coffee cups, demitasse cups, teacups, and mugs. Soda comes in 7-, 10-, and
12-ounce cans; 8-, 16-, and 32-ounce bottles; and a liter size too. Three
cans of a particular brand of soup suggest individual serving sizes of 8, 9,
and 11 ounces, respectively. A supermarket might carry upward of
25,000 items of food, all vying for your attention

*A preconceived portion size is someone else's idea of what you should eat,
based solely on what that person wants to charge you, cook for you, or serve*

you. But you must know how much *you* need—you who are 5'0" or 5'8" or 6'4" tall. At each meal, you must be able to identify the right amount of food for *you* across a crowded plate, a crowded room, or a crowded buffet table. It is your choice. This is a program, not a diet. *You* are to determine the amount of food you're adding to your plan.

Last Wednesday I met my friend Renee for lunch. She had been a participant in The Program, reached her goal weight, and kept weight off for several years. Then it began to creep up a little bit at a time so slowly, she recounted, that it was almost imperceptible. Her pants became snug where once they were loose, and she couldn't get into some of her clothes. Her waist had thickened. She could not seem to lose the 10 pounds she'd regained. Of course, bodies do change shape naturally as we get older, and we cannot expect them to remain the same as when we were eighteen years old. We can see, however, how we might be contributing to the end result.

Before we got comfortable in the Italian restaurant, a basket of garlic bread appeared on the table. Jokingly, I picked up the basket to place it on an adjoining table as I shook my head from side to side and laughingly said: "You don't want this. Do you?" I think she was too surprised to protest.

We ordered chicken—mine prepared with a little lemon and butter sauce, hers in a wine sauce with mushrooms. A platter of steamed vegetables (which we'd chosen in lieu of salads) appeared on the table between us, as did pasta with minced garlic and olive oil.

When our lunch arrived, Renee cut big chunks of her chicken, speared large pieces of vegetable, and twirled the pasta on her fork with a soupspoon. "Do you have another appointment?" I teased as she seemed to be rushing through lunch. She admitted she did eat very quickly and finally began to mirror my slower actions, putting her fork down and sipping water between bites while we conversed for well over an hour. When we were finished, there was one chicken breast left on each of our plates, more than half the vegetables, and almost all the pasta.

Since we'd last met, her lifestyle had dramatically changed: she'd gotten married, moved to the suburbs, and changed careers. After a mastectomy and chemotherapy, she was thrown into early menopause,

which she suspected had contributed to her inability to lose weight. After listening to her dilemma for an hour, I found that she had also
stopped doing some of the things that had helped her lose weight in the
first place: keeping a log (too busy), weighing regularly (too depressing),
eating cereal for breakfast instead of grabbing a bagel and coffee (too
rushed). Even with those realities, however, there were still many techniques of which she needed reminding, such as slowing down, watching
the number of items in each meal, and keeping an eye on portion size.

"Did you have enough?" I asked as we paid the check.

"Surprisingly, yes," she acknowledged.

"And we still had a nice time even though we left some food on our
plates?" I asked.

"I can't wait until we do it again," she said.

We hugged goodbye, satisfied but not stuffed.

Sam looked wide-eyed at my examples of suggested portion sizes: 4
ounces of potato. Ditto the size of containers of tuna fish and coleslaw on
the desk between us.

"I eat twice—maybe three times—that amount," he laughed.

"Do you think that's why you weigh 32 pounds more than you want
to?" I asked.

"I'll be hungry," he insisted without answering my question. "And
that looks like such a small amount of food," he said still staring at the
portion size examples.

"It's three-quarters of a pound of food," I stated, "but look how
you're projecting something that might or might not happen and we're
just sitting here in my office. You really don't know if it's going to be
enough or not unless you try," I cautioned him.

"I know. I know. But I just know it won't be enough," he continued.

"You're 15 pounds lighter than you were a few weeks ago. Is this correct?" I asked.

"Yes," he answered.

"Do you really miss all the food you obviously didn't eat?" I asked.

"Hell, yes. I'm hungry all the time," he insisted.

"Three hundred and sixty-five days a year, twenty-four hours a day?"
I questioned, in the most sweeping, exaggerated way I could muster.

"Well, maybe not *all* the time," he conceded.

"Are there any satisfying meals or good days when you're not hungry all the time?" I asked.

"I guess," he said.

"Do you think some of this hunger could be stress related?" I inquired.

"Probably a lot of it. I'm a very intense person," he acknowledged.

"So is it possible that you're not always actually hungry?" I went on.

"That's possible," he admitted.

"All I'm asking," I continued, "is that you *try* a more uniform portion size and see what happens."

"I'll keep an open mind," he said, and smiled.

Julie sits before me on a cool, damp August morning. Her pretty sandy blonde hair is the color of a schoolgirl's, yet she is a divorced mother, a grandmother, and the survivor of a stroke.

Tumbling from her lips, one after the other, are positive stories. I ordered an All-Vegetable Meal in an Italian restaurant; for the last three weeks, I've only eaten when I was hungry; I haven't had diet soda in four weeks; I had egg foo young (the Chinese version of a vegetable omelette) without gravy. She looked at me for approval.

"Gravy is okay," I smiled, "as long as it's on the side and you dip, don't drown." But, I continued, "How many pancakes did you eat?"

She nodded, a click of recognition in her eyes. She didn't answer, but we both knew three pancakes is the usual portion of egg foo young served in a Chinese restaurant, and she had eaten all three pancakes. I had not yet discussed portion size with her, but on some level, no matter how subconscious the knowledge, no matter how much in denial, she knew *(you all know)* that three pancakes is more than you need at any meal. She nodded again. I knew she knew, and she knew I knew she knew.

"But I ordered it," she continued. "Wasn't that good?" she begged for approval.

"That was very good," I agreed.

Lenny and Rhonda, a husband and wife, told stories of how they prepared the same amount of food for themselves as they used to prepare when their kids were living at home. Since the kids had been out of the house for years and had kids of their own, there were always leftovers in the Lenny and Rhonda household, but not for long. Every evening, they would consume these leftovers bite by bite and swallow by swallow, with a pick pick here and a pick pick there whenever they were in the kitchen.

"Those leftovers call my name . . . from the living room," Lenny laughed.

"And we never know when the kids might drop in," Rhonda quickly added.

"How often do they drop in without calling?" I asked.

"I guess they don't really," she acknowledged.

She told me that, for some reason, she and her husband continued to purchase, prepare, serve, and eat dinner for four almost every day. She also acknowledged they had both gained a lot of weight.

"But I do cook fish and chicken," she mentioned, "and I even steam the vegetables. Isn't that healthy?" she asked.

"Yes it is," I acknowledged. "But if you're not burning it off, it doesn't matter how seemingly healthy something is. At the end of the day, the unused food gets converted to fat and stored."

"But we don't go to those all-you-can-eat places anymore," Lenny continued, a look of pride as well as confusion crossing his face.

"But do you ever leave food on your plate?" I asked.

They looked at each other and giggled like two teenagers on a first date.

At the beginning, almost everyone wants to know, "How much of this may I eat?" Compulsive overeaters have no boundaries since no one ever told us how to say enough, *I'm fine,* or *I'm not hungry.* We don't say no to others and we don't say no to ourselves.

- If it is put on our plates, we will eat it.

- If it is served to us, it is ours.

I've highlighted just a few Portion Size *problems:* (1) eating too fast, (2) eyes bigger than stomach, (3) eating all that is served, (4) preparing too much food. Admittedly, these are just a few examples.

In the next section, you'll find some *solutions* to your portion size problems. As you read and learn to feed the smaller person you've become, you'll stop feeding the bigger person you were.

Portion Size: The Solutions

From the first day of The Program, everyone invariably asks: "How big should the portions be? How much of this item or that should I eat? Can I eat it all?"

I don't like to talk about portion size at the first session; there are too many more important things to discuss: keeping a log, weighing twice daily, slowing down, drinking water, and numerous other assignments. There is a logbook to organize, a portable scale to buy, a great deal of information to absorb. I do think that if you eat more slowly, you'll probably leave food on your plate, eat less, and ultimately lose weight.

If you've read this far, I can now tell you that 4 ounces is a portion. Four ounces of some items is easier to identify than others. A piece of chicken, a scoop of tunafish, or a potato are obvious; a salad might consist of a bit of lettuce, two mushrooms, a strip or two of carrot, a bit of celery, and so on. Therefore, salads (or a mélange of cooked vegetables), should be thought of as a 4-ounce *clump*. This is a handful of vegetables on a flat plate. You either have a 4-ounce portion of one specific item or a 4-ounce clump. No. A piece of bread is not 4 ounces, nor is a bowl of soup, nor a piece of candy. Generally almost everything else is. Sometimes even a few bites of an item might be enough.

If you're thinking that you eat much more than the 4 ounces and are concerned the new portion sizes won't be enough, it is because in the past you may have depended on visual identification of your portion size. *Yes. That looks like enough,* you'd think. What you were really thinking is: *That amount of food looks familiar. I'm comfortable with it.* A smaller portion looks unfamiliar and you feel uncomfortable with it, but you're not comfortable with your weight, either, are you? If you try the smaller portion enough times, it too will look familiar and will become comfortable. It will satisfy.

On the other hand, every now and then when your emotional hunger is great, you might take a 4-ounce can of tuna out of the cupboard and think it doesn't look like enough. But if you prepare it with mayonnaise, possibly add a salad or any other item, it is always enough. Sometimes it's too much. Learn to separate the emotion from the food. Be consistent and patient. It takes time to achieve this new way of thinking about food.

There are several ways to approach diminishing the portion size of food.

You can:

- Buy or order less.
- Prepare less.
- Serve less.
- Eat less.

Buy Less

If you've been annotating your log, chances are you've been writing that you are leaving food over. You might also concede that smaller amounts are usually enough. The next step would be to buy or prepare less the next time. As you become a smaller person, you will realize you don't require as much food as you did when you were a bigger person, so purchase smaller portions:

- Buy potatoes that are 4 ounces. If you are cooking for more than one person, buy potatoes that can be divided into 4-ounce portions.

- Choose boneless, skinless chicken breasts in a package as close to a pound as you can find. When you arrive home, divide the package into four individual 4-ounce portions, and freeze them in separate freezer bags. Do the same with chopped meat, veal cutlets, chicken wings, fish, and other foods. Inquire of the butcher what the edible-to-bone ratio is so you can package accordingly.

- Buy tuna, salmon, smoked oysters, and sardines in individual 4-ounce tins.

- Purchase a quarter-pound of sliced turkey, or coleslaw, or anything else that can be weighed. Look at it on a plate, think about how you feel after you've eaten for 20 minutes, and acknowledge that this amount has truly satisfied you.

- Instead of looking for the bigger of anything, look for the smaller: medium eggs, smaller chickens, fruits, and vegetables.

- If you're in a restaurant, you can request an appetizer portion of a dish as your main course. Perhaps two appetizers would be a perfect meal.

- If dinner is late, consider sharing an entrée with a friend.

- Think of soup and salad as being the right amount of Food/Energy to eat before seeing a late movie. Sometimes soup by itself is the perfect amount.

- Want dessert? Purchase an individual pastry instead of an entire box, a scoop of ice cream instead of a pint, and so on. Ralph, a participant in The Program, used to say, "I only order dessert in a restaurant because in a restaurant they don't bring you the whole container, bag, or box."

Prepare Less

- Prepare a quarter of a smaller chicken the way you like it, and it will be just as satisfying as a quarter of a larger chicken. Because you are used to eating everything on your plate, it doesn't matter if an item is smaller or bigger; you will eat it. Therefore, you might as well avoid a Possible Pitfall and buy, order, prepare, and serve less in the first place.

- Put one chop (pork, veal, or lamb) on your plate, instead of two.

- Prepare or purchase a quarter-pound each of grilled chicken, tossed salad, and rice, and arrange them attractively on a plate. (If you purchase prepared food, make sure you take these foods out of the containers before eating them.) Eat slowly and thoughtfully. Put your utensils down between bites. Sip water. Cut smaller pieces, and create a 20-Minute Meal. Focus on the quantity of food. What does it look like? How do you physically feel before you eat? How do you feel when you've finished eating? Was it too much? Too little? Enough? You'll be surprised. Twelve ounces of food is three-quarters of a pound of food, and that is a generous amount of food for almost any size appetite. Maybe you only need a two-item meal—about a half pound of food.

When you've created an atmosphere in your kitchen that makes the 4-ounce portion your size, you will be able to go into the real world and when food is served, think: *How much greater in size are the portions set before me than the portions I've been eating all week, which were enough?* Leave the difference on your plate.

While I was attending a sculpture course for several years at the New School in New York City, at the beginning of each semester the new students asked the teacher how to carve an elephant. With a twinkle in his eye, our teacher would answer, "Get a block of marble, and chip away everything that doesn't look like an elephant."

Portion size is the same thing. Once you find your portion size, chip away everything that doesn't look like your portion.

If you prepare 4-ounce portion sizes at home, only to eat the chef's portion in a restaurant or Aunt Martha's portion every Friday night, you will be practicing a form of deprivation in order to binge. If you have so many exceptions to the rule, you won't have any rule. Without consistency, your body will not feel compelled to seek out the 4-ounce portion size because you won't feel uncomfortable when you eat more, and smaller portions won't seem familiar. Choosing 4-ounce portions Monday, Wednesday, and Friday and bigger portions Tuesday, Thursday, and when you're on vacation or traveling will only add to your fear that the smaller amount won't be enough. Your stomach will always stretch to accommodate any size portion. The reason to eat is not to stretch your stomach (and ultimately your body) out of shape, but to nourish your body so you'll have the energy to carry you through your daily activities.

- Package foods into single-portion sizes as soon as you bring them home, and freeze them.

- Consume 4-ounce portions again and again. When you do overeat, you'll feel discomfort—a gentle reminder that overeating doesn't feel so good.

- Although 4-ounce portions are enough, should you feel hungry later, you can always have a Fourth Meal.

- Eat enough Food/Energy at one meal to take you to the next (or in the case of dinner, to bed). It is not necessary to eat oversized amounts of food at one meal because you might have missed a previous meal.

Uniformity of portion size (balance) is important. If you have big items at one meal and small ones at another, your mind and body won't know which habit you're trying to create. If one item—for example, a salad—is oversized and everything else on the plate is smaller, you'll feel a sense of deprivation. You'll want all items to be the size of your salad. Count it as two salads (salad, salad), plus chicken and potato: four items of food, not three. Remember: It doesn't matter if it's a cookie or a carrot. It all adds up. (See Example One.)

Example One

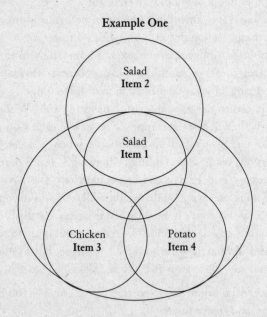

Take a chance and get comfortable with uniform 4-ounce portion sizes. If you eat slowly, it will be enough.

The next example, noodle soup, was on Suzi's suggested Meal Plan.

She decided that she needed a protein at the meal. She had chicken breasts in the freezer and decided to add chicken to the soup.

Perhaps half the soup and half the chicken breast will make a satisfying meal without increasing its original volume. (See Example Two.)

Example Two

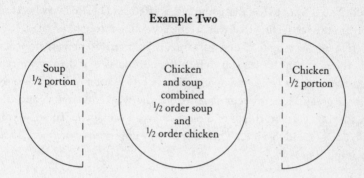

The portion of a bottle of wine is a family-style portion as opposed to one glass, which would be à la carte style. If you order one bottle and there are two of you, each receives a half-bottle, which you or the waiter will continue to pour until it is empty. Three or more people at the table? There is always the possibility that someone will want to order a second bottle. The more glasses of wine you drink as part of the meal, the more out of balance the meal becomes. A second glass of wine makes it a multiple—wine, wine. If you're losing weight with an abundance of one item over another, you're probably not getting as much nutrition as you would from a wider variety of food choices. And because alcohol causes lack of resolve, you'll end up drinking and eating more than you planned.

I've discussed the balance of portions on each plate so that the items are uniform. One item may look small on the plate, but if it is satisfying, then it is enough; that is your portion size. Four ounces of sliced turkey is visually quite different from 4 ounces of shrimp.

You might be accustomed to some items being bigger than others, such as salads, steaks, and baked potatoes.

A salad used to contain lettuce, tomato, cucumber, and perhaps a slice or two of carrot and celery. Now, many salads contain olives, croutons, peppers, sprouts, mushrooms, celery, and other items. You might think it is acceptable to feel stuffed and bloated because it is only salad, or that soup contains so much water it can't be equal to a potato, for example. If you allow your stomach to be stretched out of shape with large amounts of food believed to be low in calories and you get comfortable feeling stuffed, when low-calorie food is not available, you'll eat higher-calorie food. You'll want to feel that same full, stuffed, and bloated way because you are used to feeling that way from eating those troughs of salad.

If you're leaving food on your plate, it is a signal to prepare or order less the next time. Once you reduce the portion size, it does not mean that two months from now when you are on vacation or on a business trip or going home to your parents' for the weekend, you should increase your portion. If half of a piece of bread is okay on Tuesday, you don't want to double it on Thursday by consuming an entire piece. (See Example Three.)

Example Three

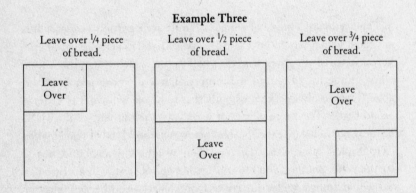

Leave over ¼ piece of bread.

Leave over ½ piece of bread.

Leave over ¾ piece of bread.

It means that no matter where you are, your portion size is the reduced amount with which you were comfortable while in your *Home Base*.

As you get in the habit of choosing 4 ounces across the board, you will find yourself filling up that much sooner and leaving food over more often than in the past. You are a smaller person, and it will seem natural for you to buy and prepare food for the smaller person you've become.

Serve Fewer Items

If you bring home prepared food, serve yourself first, then package and freeze the leftovers before sitting down to eat. You'll be less likely to pick if there are no visible leftovers. If food is instantly available on your kitchen counter, you're likely to think: "Oh, well. It's only one more shrimp, one more piece of broccoli," and the leftovers won't be left over.

- Reduce the number of items at each meal, if appropriate. If you've been having two for breakfast and not losing weight, try some one-item meals. If you've been ordering two or three items for lunch, try a bowl of soup and a salad one day or different two-item meals for another few days. Do the same for dinner. Experiment.

- Serve one plate per person, rather than family style. If family style is necessary, leave the platters and bowls in the kitchen or on a sideboard, where you can tell everyone, "There's plenty in the other room," but you won't be tempted by having to stare at them all through dinner.

- Order à la carte rather than the prix fixe meal, which usually contains courses you wouldn't normally be ordering.

Overeating is overeating. Watch the portion size of salads, vegetables, and beverages, as well as desserts, breads, alcohol, and High-End Protein.

Many of us are used to watching the portion size of things we consider high in calories such as dessert and bread, and then think that we can have unlimited quantities of salads, vegetables, and low-calorie beverages. This type of erroneous thinking hasn't worked. If you have a wide variety of foods, sometimes salad and sometimes potato, and they are both the same size portion, your stomach will get used to a certain amount of volume. Anything over that amount, whether high or low in calories, will make you feel uncomfortable. Sometimes dessert and sometimes a cup of tea will achieve the same result.

Say it out loud, *More is not better; it is only more.*

Holiday, travel, rain, loneliness, stress, or boredom does not mean second portions tonight. Find another hobby.

There is no such thing as little, crumb, small, just, tiny, or trivial. If you swallowed it, you ate it, and it all adds up.

Eat Less

A lot of eating is done because it's there, or it looked good, smelled good, or it was easily available.

No matter what my frame of mind, I don't believe I have ever really had willpower or self-control, or I would not have gained 50 pounds in the first place. If sometimes I don't eat bread from the basket on a restaurant table, or if I don't finish a box of cookies in one sitting, one day, or even one week, it is just a coincidence. I live alone and will eventually finish the box or bag. So it is important that I remain mindful of my food needs and buy, prepare, and serve the appropriate amount. It is important I order the correct amount when dining out too. In that way, no matter where I am, I will eat the right amount of food for me.

Plan ahead which category of food, the Number of Items in each meal, and whether to eat a Filler. This will help you buy or order (prepare and serve) the necessary amounts of food for the meal you're about to eat.

When I'm particularly stressed or tired, it is sometimes tempting to surrender to the urges and compulsions of my disease, so I try to be prepared for Possible Pitfalls as early in each day as possible by anticipating and planning ahead.

I eat less now because I don't require as much food as I once did. It doesn't seem like less, or small, or even not enough. It is my portion size, and it is fine physically. If sometimes it doesn't seem like enough emotionally, I know if I'm looking to prepare more food than I need, it's because I am trying to distract myself from some feeling of discomfort. It could be anxiety, stress, fatigue, or a combination of many things.

As I write this, I am very tired. It is very late. It is the beginning of a Labor Day weekend, and I've got deadlines I must meet. I know I'm not hungry, but I am thinking about doing anything other than work on this chapter. Food is available as something to do. It's not that I could or would clean a closet at 3:00 A.M. But I don't act on these feelings. I just acknowledge them. If I take a short break and do something else, I know the moment will pass.

If you are consistent with your portion size, you will get comfortable with this thinking, too. You will realize the new amount will be enough. Sometimes it will even seem like too much.

Nut and Seed Sheet Commentary

The Program does not count calories, but it might be helpful to know that 4 ounces of nuts, seeds, popcorn, or potato chips is equal to, *or more than,* three meals, each containing a portion of chicken, broccoli, and potato.

Three plates of food, three meals, do not contain as many calories as a handful of nuts.

Three chicken-vegetable-potato meals, with all the chewing, crunching, and enjoyment, *or* a handful of (Finger Foods, alert. Alert!) nuts, seeds, popcorn, or potato chips? The choice is yours.

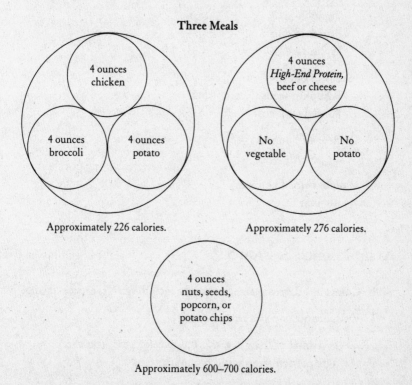

Three Meals

4 ounces chicken

4 ounces broccoli

4 ounces potato

Approximately 226 calories.

4 ounces *High-End Protein,* beef or cheese

No vegetable

No potato

Approximately 276 calories.

4 ounces nuts, seeds, popcorn, or potato chips

Approximately 600–700 calories.

A woman tells me how her seventeen-year-old daughter sprinkles Sesame seeds on her salad. She asks, "Why can't *I*?"

I tell her we are compulsive eaters. We don't know from sprinkle. We only know, buy a pound, eat a pound.

Nuts (4 ounces)	Calories
Almonds	678
Beechnuts	644
Brazil nuts	742
Butternuts	713
Cashew nuts	639
Hickory nuts	767
Macadamia nuts	784
Peanuts	640
Pecans	779
Pignolia	626
Pistachio nuts	674
Walnuts	713

Seeds (4 ounces)	
Pumpkin seeds	627
Sunflower seeds	635

Popcorn (4 ounces)	
air popped	640

Potato chips (4 ounces)	
Regular	640

Assignments: Session 5

1. Continue all previous assignments including: Never stop trying.

2. Evaluate portion size before eating.

   a. Is it smaller than it was a few weeks ago? You are. The portion size should be smaller too.

   b. Is it growing?

   c. Is it enough?

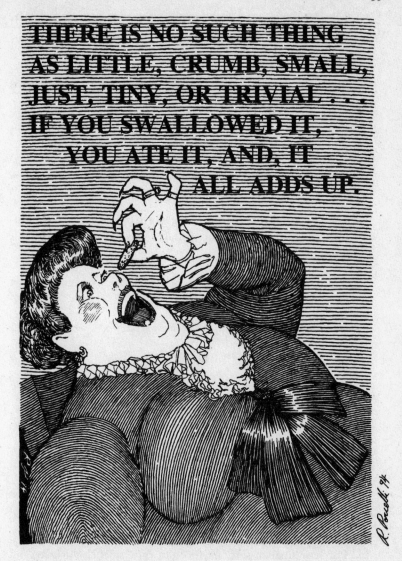

THERE IS NO SUCH THING
AS LITTLE, CRUMB, SMALL,
JUST, TINY, OR TRIVIAL . . .
IF YOU SWALLOWED IT,
YOU ATE IT, AND, IT
ALL ADDS UP.

3. Don't wait to eat until you're famished, starved, or ravenous.

4. Don't ever eat so much that you're stuffed or bloated. Remember
    to drink water.

5. Don't eat so much at one meal that you're not hungry for the next.

6. Wear a belt with a buckle whenever eating, whenever possible. If your clothing is of the loose kind, wear a thin belt under your clothing.

7. Make sure your nutritional needs are met before choosing foods from the top or bottom of the Meal Parameters list.

8. During a meal, ask: Am I still hungry? And if not, leave something over.

9. Plan what you're going to eat, and buy only what is on your list—no aisle cruising, no menu cruising.

10. Plan the Number of Items you're going to consume. Use repatterning techniques to relax yourself while getting comfortable with this assignment.

11. Plan Fillers in advance of each meal: bread *or* beverage *or* dessert *or* alcohol—one of four or none.

12. Serve French style rather than family style.

13. Buy à la carte, not a prix fixe meal.

14. Annotate your log with portion size (e.g., *I used to eat more and now I'm eating less, but it is enough*).

15. When the appropriate time has come:

    a. Throw out one big item of clothing so you won't grow back into that size again.

    b. Try on clothes in a smaller size.

    c. Acknowledge you are a smaller person.

16. Purchase smaller portions, medium eggs, smaller chickens, and smaller fruits and vegetables.

17. Order, buy, and purchase a little less of everything, including The Fillers.

18. Package foods into single-portion sizes upon arriving home, and freeze them. If you bring home prepared food, serve yourself

first, then package and freeze the leftovers before sitting down to eat.

19. Overeating is overeating. Watch portion sizes of salads, vegetables, and beverages, as well as desserts, breads, alcohol, and High-End Protein.

20. Overeating doesn't change the outcome of anything except your waistline and self-esteem. Feed a smaller person.

21. More is not better. It is only more.

22. Holiday, travel, rain, loneliness, stress, or boredom does not mean second portions tonight. Find another hobby.

23. Leave one bite of food on your plate each day—each meal, if possible.

24. There is no such thing as little, crumb, small, just, tiny, or trivial. If you swallowed it, you ate it, and it all adds up.

25. Keep a running list of all the things you *do* accomplish each day, including all things that have improved since the first week.

26. What three things can you do this week for each assignment you've not yet conquered?

    a. _____

    b. _____

    c. _____

    Use a combination of physical/mental/verbal/relaxing repatterning techniques for best results. When a difficult moment arises, move the food, or move yourself.

27. Write a Meal Plan of your own this week, and *try* to make it happen. If you'd rather not write your own, use any one of the four in the book.

28. Review notes daily. If this is not happening, make an appointment with yourself to do it. Even fifteen minutes a day can make a difference.

29. Cheer yourself on rather than beat yourself up. Maintain a positive attitude, and you will get positive results.

30. Rewrite these assignments into your logbook.

31. Repeat often to yourself, "I want to weigh _____ pounds; I can do it!"

32. Review your notes daily or more often.

Quantum Leaps

Review/Rate Your Progress

Date _____

Weight at the first session _____
This morning _____
Plus / Minus Difference _____ pounds

Enter 1, 2, 3, or 4 for each item in the list, according to this key:

4 = Part of your life and comfortable
3 = Aware and trying
2 = Improving, but could be better
1 = Holding onto old habits

1. I am aware of food, weight, and measurements daily. ____

2. I slow down, put food on a plate, use utensils when eating. ____

3. I get a variety of cereals, All-Vegetable Meals, and soup meals. ____

4. I drink eight to ten (or more) glasses of water, hot or cold, daily. ____

5. I eat only when I am hungry. ____

6. I stop eating when I am no longer hungry. ____

7. I eat bread *or* beverage *or* dessert *or* alcohol— one of four or none. ____

8. I know the Meal Parameters and Guidelines and use them. ___

9. I count Fillers each day and total Fillers each week. ___

10. I use a Meal Plan each day. ___

11. I consume five or six items daily (with an occasional four-item or seven-item day), with one, two, three, or four at dinner; one, two, or three at lunch; and one or two at breakfast. ___

12. I choose a uniform portion size for all items. ___

13. I leave food on my plate each day. ___

14. I acknowledge strong new habits as they become more comfortable. ___

15. I am aware of habits that need work. ___

16. I put an action plan in writing to change things that need work. ___

17. I remember the reasons I want to reach my weight-loss goal. ___

18. I remember the reasons I want to be thinner. ___

19. I remember the negatives of overeating. ___

20. I remember the negatives of overweight. ___

21. I enjoy the positives of eating the right amount for me. ___

22. I enjoy the positives of being a smaller person. ___

23. I am aware of habits being formed, old ones disappearing. ___

24. I review notes daily and adjust actions accordingly. ___

25. I keep on keeping on, and never stop trying. ___

Total ___

Rewrite into your logbook for daily review.

There are a possible 100 points. Most of you are able to order exactly what you want, in amounts you want, to be eaten when you want. This occurs approximately 80 to 95 percent of the time. But even if you're at a command-performance dinner at midnight and the main course is roast beef with a side order of lamb chops, *you still don't have to say yes to every course, and you don't have to finish everything on your plate.*

Where you rated your progress as 1 or 2, enter those items on a *Needs Work* page. Review your notes as usual, and spend a little more time on the items that need work.

Positive Thinking

Following are comments in response to my question, "What are you doing now that you had not done before exposure to The Program?" Add your own favorites, using the phrases *I am* or *I have,* as if it is already so.

> "I am a slender person, and I do the things a slender person does."

> "I am thinking there is always another meal. The one I'm eating is not the Last Supper."

> "I am choosing my thoughts as carefully as I choose my foods."

> "I am choosing to put only healthy foods into my body."

> "I feed the smaller person I am."

> "I am a thin person because I choose to be thin."

> "I am using water as a distraction from boredom."

> "I think twice before eating."

> "I am a thinner person, and I do not need as much food as I used to need."

> "I am a happy person and do not need food to make me happy."

"I am a busy person and do not need food to occupy my time."

"I have a full life. I don't need my stomach to be full."

"I have control of my food. It does not control me."

"The moments will pass whether I eat or not."

"No one else cares whether I say *no, thank you.*"

"Breaking habits is like cleaning house. You do an area in a room first. Then you finish the room, and then you complete the house. And then you start over again."

Quantum Leaps I Have Jumped

I'm a failure.

I cheated.

I'm so bad.

I binged.

I lost weight and celebrated with an entire cake.

I have no willpower.

I have no self-control.

I'm a weak person.

I can't do anything right.

I'm bad.

I do everything wrong.

The above declarations are remnants of a diet mentality—if *I can't do it perfectly, I won't do it at all*—from which you are striving desperately to rid yourself. You might have an unending habit of pointing out, reliving, keeping alive, and always repeating to yourself or anyone who will listen how bad you are. This type of thinking does not work. You only hear *I'm bad, I cheated, I failed.* Sometimes these thoughts are a self-fulfilling prophecy.

Many overweight people are in the habit of berating themselves for the slightest indiscretion, the implication being: "In order to lose weight, I have to be perfect." Of course, all you can ever hope for is to do the very best you can under the circumstances. And if you're able to accomplish that, you cannot beat yourself up. The new way to think is: *Whatever I did, I did less of it, stopped sooner, and don't do it as frequently as I once did.*

All those instances when you thought you blew it were merely you bumping into stimuli you had not anticipated, and you reverted to your previous practiced, familiar, almost involuntary behavior. If you do nothing to change your conditioned responses to these encounters, the old way is the only one you will ever know. By continuing the old way, you reinforce that old behavior once again, locking it in even more tightly.

Repatterning techniques are designed to chip away and neutralize your practiced behaviors until they are different. You don't have to succeed 100 percent of the time. It is the efforts and attempts to change, the baby steps that, when repeated again and again become the *Quantum Leaps.* To reinforce new habits until they become almost involuntary, create a Quantum Leaps list of your own. By acknowledging the successful outcome of an assignment—something you're doing now that you've never been able to do before—you begin to make it a solid, concrete habit.

To focus on the positives—the Quantum Leaps you have jumped— begin a page in your logbook titled Quantum Leaps I Have Jumped and write a beginning list of fifteen leaps you've taken since beginning your weight-loss program. Think about things of a physical, mental nature with regard to the foods you have chosen, the way you feel about yourself, your new weight, and your new awareness. One Quantum Leap might be that you leave the table before you finish all the food on your plate, or brush your teeth instead of pouring your usual cup of coffee at four o'clock, and it's all okay—better than okay.

A Quantum Leap might be that you're wearing clothes you haven't fit into in years or traveling with your scale—something you're doing now that you were not doing before exposure to The Program. By capturing these Quantum Leaps in writing, each time you review your notes, you'll be reminded that you did these things once and you can do them again.

To help you get started I've listed some other people's Quantum Leaps. I encourage you to capture some of these for your own list. Conversely, if you happen across a Quantum Leap on this list that you're not yet doing but would like to, you might enter it on your Needs Work page.

Other People's Quantum Leaps

I eat only when I'm hungry.

I am more in control and less out of control.

I don't plan to overeat.

Breaking away from old food combinations.

Dipping salad dressing rather than drowning my salad.

No candy in the movies, and I don't miss it.

No popcorn in the movies, and nobody died.

Not eating except when I'm hungry. *That* is amazing!

Breakfast without bread is fine.

I keep a detailed log of everything I eat.

No calorie counting.

Learned to say *no, thank you* and mean it.

Reached my goal weight.

Food is less important.

Filling up sooner.

I can cross my legs.

The scale is my friend.

Reviewing notes is comforting.

Making choices rather than being a victim.

Enjoying water instead of most other beverages.

No upset stomach or indigestion.

Not opening and closing the refrigerator door.

I like eating with utensils, not fingers.

Anticipating and planning ahead.

Breakfast feels good.

Bringing the right foods into the house.

Enjoying compliments about weight loss.

When I look in the mirror, I see a difference.

Traveling with a scale.

Emerging hipbones and cheekbones.

Able to think more clearly.

Sharper, more creative, and more productive.

More effort to eat green vegetables.

No diet soda or diet products; better than okay.

Variety is more satisfying than volume.

Diminished frequency of Fillers is fine.

Choosing less High-End Protein, including cheese.

Making healthier food choices.

Motivated to move around more.

Not stuffed all the time after eating.

Choosing bread *or* beverage *or* dessert *or* alcohol—one of four or none.

I look and feel younger.

Better sleep patterns.

More self-respect.

Found and enjoy thick soup.

Found and enjoy All-Vegetable Meals.

More 20-Minute Meals than not.

Noticeable savings of money.

Less difficulty tying shoelaces.

One- and two-item meals are okay.

No noshing.

Not feeling deprived.

Not feeling I'm dieting.

Able to eat in any restaurant and no one knows I'm doing anything special.

Not afraid of food. It's just food.

No bingeing.

No more mindless eating.

I feel lighter and more buoyant.

Proud to have my picture taken.

Weight off my mind as well as body.

Desire to clothes-shop again.

I leave food on my plate and don't miss it.

Taking care of myself.

It's a relief to be in control.

Increased consciousness and mindfulness.

Enjoying meals without overeating.

Less self-hatred.

I put down fork many times during each meal.

Separating food and emotion.

Less frequent headaches.

Not displacing anger or anxiety with food.

Making and taking the time to eat.

Guilt-free desserts.

Relaxing and eating more slowly.

Tasting my food, not just gobbling it.

Aware that my new portion size is fine.

I'm feeding a smaller person.

Finding out that salads are also food.

I don't need to eat to socialize.

I don't need alcohol to have a nice time.

I can buy normal-sized clothes.

Threw out large pair of pants.

Clothes are hanging on me.

Filling up sooner.

I don't feel helpless anymore.

I am happier with myself.

Getting by on less food.

Increased self-esteem.

Not using food when I am bored or in pain.

I look better, feel better, and sex is better.

I have more stamina and can dance without immediately becoming tired.

I can endure stress without resorting to food.

Enjoying slower meals.

My bathing suit is too big. I am no longer a size 16 or W.

I look in the mirror, and I like what I see.

I feel powerful.

I feel confident in public about my appearance.

I am close to my college weight—eighteen years ago.

I look and feel younger and more energetic.

Hot water really *is* satisfying.

My energy level has improved.

I am bolder about asking for what I want—both food-wise and otherwise.

I enjoy eating more slowly—not wolfing it all down.

I'm learning to be less hurried in general—a stress reliever.

I can stay awake driving without coffee and candy.

My watch slides down my arm.

Better posture.

Smaller stomach now.

Smaller than my spouse!

Fish has entered my life.

I don't hang out in kitchen. I find other things to do.

I'm not as depressed.

I'm eating a lot more vegetables.

My small jeans are getting big!

Knee-high's don't stop my circulation.

A spring in my step.

I can do anything.

I can tie my shoelace without causing internal bleeding.

My wraparound robe actually wraps around.

I am proud of myself.*

Add any Quantum Leaps to your list that you remembered while reading of others' accomplishments. Number your Quantum Leaps. You'll notice, as you review your notes each day, that many new ways of thinking and acting have become habits you can put on your list. Always add a few extra blank numbers at the end of your list to remind you that this is a work in progress. You should always be striving to add new Quantum Leaps to your list. Throw away even *one* cookie the first time, and you have one more Quantum Leap. Then each time you review your Quantum Leaps list, you'll think, *I did that once, and it was comfortable. I could do it again.*

One of my most treasured Quantum Leaps was learning how to put my fork down between bites. I realized that mealtime was not marathon time and that I wasn't on my way to a fire. Another big Quantum Leap I've jumped is taking the time to prepare and eat hot cereal for breakfast; a meal I had always considered unimportant is now very enjoyable. I often have hot cereal for lunch or dinner if I didn't have it for breakfast that day. That was important on several levels: the enjoyment of a whole-grain cereal and, while preparing it, the feeling that I am doing something nice for myself. The satisfying taste and texture made me realize that every meal need not contain a salad, protein, vegetable, starch, dessert, and coffee. One-item meals can be very enjoyable.

One participant's favorite Quantum Leap follows:

> I love to swim, but I haven't set foot in a pool in twenty
> years. A few years ago, a cousin asked me if I wanted
> to rent a villa on the Italian coast for the summer. I
> always made some excuse to avoid disrobing. I was

*You should be proud because when all is said and done, you are out there alone and are doing all of this yourself.

terrified of romping around the Riviera in shorts and a
t-shirt. This year we're doing it. And do you know
what? I'm actually looking forward to it. I'm down
forty pounds, have been taking care of myself, and am
proud of the way I look.

I went to an antique store recently and bought
something for myself because I'm finally accepting the
fact that I'm worth it. In the past, I would have bought
the item as a gift for someone else or not bought it at
all. When I decided to buy it for myself because I
thought I deserved it, it was very emotional.

I work for a very posh clothing store and not only
can I afford fashionable clothes, I also get an employee
discount, so there's no reason for me not to dress beau-
tifully. But when I was heavier—I've lost 40 pounds—
I looked only for clothes to cover my girth. People
cannot believe I hid all the weight, but I did—under
vests, behind eye-distracting ties, and dark-colored
suits. I'm an expert at camouflage. It's my business.

The weight loss has changed my life. I feel so much
more confident, more outgoing. No one could ever
understand how the weight affected my life. (*Bob J.*)

What is *your* most important Quantum Leap?

Body Image

What do you look like? How big (or small) are you? How tall (or short)?
How much do you weigh?

When I ask participants how much they weighed when they were
teenagers, I hear this lament: They thought they were very heavy, but
when they look at those old photos now, they realize they weighed 130
pounds, a weight they'd be thrilled to weigh today.

To feel comfortable feeding the smaller person you've become, be
honest about your weight, silhouette, image, and self. You might be hav-

ing a hard time giving up the big person image with which you are so comfortable. It is, after all, familiar, possibly since childhood. Unhappiness about weight is part of the web of habits created to distract us from other painful thoughts and feelings.

How you looked as a child is how you might now see yourself. If you were a thin child, you might still see yourself as thin, even though you've gained weight. And if you were a heavy child, you might find it hard to believe you're thinner, even though you've lost weight. Getting comfortable with the new smaller you is a matter of taking a few steps to reinforce a body image more closely related to the new reality.

Buy a full-length mirror, if you don't already have one.

Step one: Undress and look in it daily.

Step two: Repeat step one.

Just like keeping a food diary or drinking ten glasses of water or weighing yourself twice daily, looking in your full-length mirror must be part of the structure of your program. A mirror jolts you out of your weight-loss complacency.

Another assignment of awareness is to get your picture taken. Take out your camera, get a roll of film, and have a friend snap shots of you sitting, standing, front view, side view, back view, standing straight, and bending over. Smile, frown, pose, and change outfits. Wear slacks, suits, skirts, dresses, cover-ups, and fitted clothing. Wear nothing. A photograph is the moment in time when you know your weight problems and successes are no longer a secret. Others know you've gained (or lost) weight.

When I was 50 pounds heavier, I dressed differently. I tended to buy shapeless overblouses, A-line dresses and skirts, and generally baggy clothing. I thought of myself as young and thin, so I was really startled to see a photograph of me looking old and fat. One winter day while waiting for a bus and even more padded than usual with extra sweaters and a quilted jacket, someone asked me how many months pregnant I was. I was not.

When I lost the weight, however, I again saw myself in a photograph with a friend I'd always considered half my size. I'd thought of myself as much bigger than my friend, even though the photograph showed clearly I was actually much smaller.

The late comedian Selma Diamond told a wonderful story about shopping in a clothing store on Lincoln Road, a street with cachet in Miami Beach, Florida. "As I tried on a dress, the saleswoman oohed and aahed while she lingered in the doorway of the dressing room," Diamond recounted. The saleswoman said, "That dress was made for you." "Yes," Diamond deadpanned, "but you made it too small."

Weigh, measure, and go shopping. Try on all kinds of clothing in a smaller size to corroborate what the scale says. You might feel heavy one day because of water retention, possibly from overly salty food, but if the scale is down or you slide into a smaller-sized skirt, shirt, slacks, panties, belt, bra, or ring, it's because you're smaller.

Experiment with colors that are brighter and clothing in a different style from those worn by the heavier you. A lot of people who have lost weight are thrilled to see themselves wearing a belt for the first time in years, buckling a belt a notch tighter, or wearing tuck-ins rather than overshirts. Get your hair styled; shave off your moustache. Dress like the smaller person you've become.

Kirsten lost a fair amount of weight and followed an assignment to buy one new article of clothing in a smaller size. She paraded around my office pretending to model her new dress. I applauded; she did look terrific. "It's a size 8," she exclaimed incredulously. I beamed for her. She deserved it. And then her smile faded, as if she couldn't believe *she* was wearing a size 8. "Of course, it's not *really* a size 8," she said. "It's cut very big." Yet all the evidence pointed to the fact that when she was 20 pounds heavier, she could not have fit into that size 8 dress even if it was cut big.

You weigh more than you want to weigh all over, and that is how you will lose it. It will happen gradually and subtly and won't always be noticeable, so don't expect extreme, daily, dramatic changes.

Weight loss becomes obvious when you've lost anywhere from 5 to 15 pounds. With me, no one noticed until I'd lost about 25 or 30 pounds because I continued to wear those tent-like cover-ups.

Many of the clothes in your closet might be brand new, because as soon as you bought them, your weight increased; some clothes might even have the price tags still attached. Try them on. You might need to tailor them to fit. You might decide to give your clothes to charity. Clean your closets so that everything in them fits. Then you won't grow back into those bigger sizes. When everything fits perfectly and you eat more than you need, you'll feel the discomfort. If you continually eat more than you need and wear elastic-waisted clothing, your waistbands will stretch to accommodate any amount of food, and the discomfort won't be obvious.

When you put on something new in a smaller size that fits, people will notice the fit or the color and corroborate the fact that *you look marvelous!* Compliments are the best encouragement for you to continue feeding the smaller you. Sometimes, however, it is the inclination of a person with low self-esteem to neutralize a compliment by saying something like, "Yes, but [the words of an addict] I have so much more to lose." By doing this, you're wiping out all that you have accomplished. If you don't take responsibility for the baby steps you have achieved, and don't acknowledge you really are a smaller person and are the one responsible for having become a smaller person, you'll never feed the smaller person you've become. When someone tells you, you look great, say: *Thank you.* Period. Don't say *thank you* and then take it away with a *yes, but, it's not really a size 8; it's cut big.* Just say: *Thank you.* Period.

Suppose you have a pair of slacks or a pretty brown shirt that you've worn through a 20-pound weight gain; only you know the nuance of the fit as it moves from comfortably big to uncomfortably small. Friends, of course, know only that you're wearing the pretty brown shirt again. If you go through life reinforcing destructive behavior by pointing out your imperfections, people will only notice your imperfections (big stomach or wide hips, for example). They won't see your handsome or pretty face.

When I was 50 pounds heavier, I looked down and saw breasts and belly and thighs not quite the shape and girth I wanted them to be. Fifty pounds lighter, I look down and see the same body parts. I know my body is 50 pounds lighter, but it sort of looks and feels the same to me. I do know, however, my daily weight, clothing size, ring size, belt size, and shoe sizes are all telling me I am a smaller person. When you lose your weight, you have to acknowledge the weight loss and feed the smaller person you've become. The smaller you doesn't have to eat as frequently as before and doesn't require as much food.

When I had just lost the weight, I went to a casual clothing shop and stood in line at the checkout counter waiting to buy a pair of elastic-waisted pants. A woman standing behind me in line told me I had such a cute figure that I could wear anything, including the pants I planned on buying. I proudly told her I had just lost 50 pounds. "Then don't buy those elastic-waisted pants," she whispered. "You'll only grow back into them and gain all the weight back." *She is absolutely correct,* I thought. I put the pants on the counter and fled the store, thanking her over my shoulder as I raced toward the street. Do your clothes fit because the material stretches? Have you grown into your jogging pants?

Health note: When you've lost (or gained) a few pounds, whether from overeating or pregnancy (even if you don't carry the baby to term or have a cesarean), get your diaphragm refitted. You lose inches inside as well as out.

Summary (rewrite into your logbook for daily reviews).

- Get photographs taken of yourself.

- Weigh yourself morning and evening.

- Look at yourself in a full-length mirror. Buy new items that fit.

- Make sure all your clothing fits properly, especially when you arrive at your weight-loss destination. Have your diaphragm refitted. Size your rings.

- Wear a belt with a buckle whenever eating, whenever possible. If you like oversized clothing, wear a thin belt under your clothes.

- Remind yourself you are smaller (mental repatterning).

- Get rid of the old slacks, the big sacks, the tents and tarpaulins, the *boombalotti* dresses.

- Find a tailor, or do it yourself, but alter your clothes to reflect the new smaller you. Those of you with relatively big weight fluctuations have several wardrobe sizes hanging in the closet. Get all your clothes to fit properly; get rid of the rest.

- Don't ever eat so much that you're stuffed or bloated.

- Throw away the biggest article of clothing you own. Tear it up and march it out to the curb, or at the very least, throw it into the trash. What you're telling yourself symbolically is, *I'll never grow into that size again!*

- Go to your closet or a store, and try on clothes in a smaller size that fits. Begin wearing one new smaller article of clothing every few weeks.

- Walk tall. You lost weight. You are a smaller person. Be proud!

- Keep a photo of a thin you visible. Look at it daily.

Which body image do you want to convey to others?

Comprehensive Review

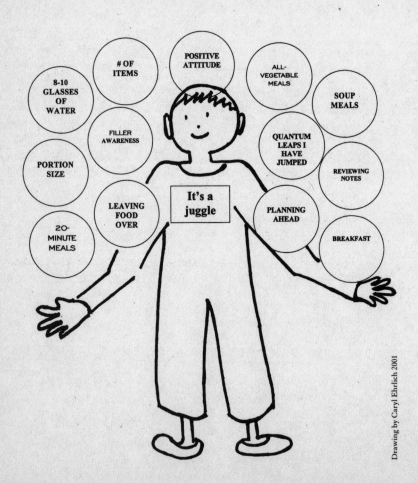

8-10
GLASSES
OF
WATER

OF
ITEMS

POSITIVE
ATTITUDE

ALL-
VEGETABLE
MEALS

SOUP
MEALS

FILLER
AWARENESS

QUANTUM
LEAPS I
HAVE
JUMPED

PORTION
SIZE

REVIEWING
NOTES

LEAVING
FOOD
OVER

It's a
juggle

PLANNING
AHEAD

20-
MINUTE
MEALS

BREAKFAST

Drawing by Caryl Ehrlich 2001

Review of Previous Assignments

Date _____

Weight at the first session? _____
This morning? _____
Plus / Minus Difference _____ pounds.

	More Often Than Not	Try to Make It Happen	Seldom or Never Accomplished
1. I keep a detailed log of food.	___	___	___
2. I weigh daily A.M. and P.M.	___	___	___
3. I review assignments and Needs Work page daily.	___	___	___
4. I anticipate my daily food needs and plan accordingly.	___	___	___
5. Before consuming any food I ask, *Am I hungry or what?*	___	___	___
6. If I am not hungry, I ascertain why I'm thinking of eating.	___	___	___
7. If I am hungry, I create a 20-minute relaxing meal.	___	___	___
8. When eating, I put food on a plate and eat with utensils.	___	___	___
9. I eat from the middle of the Meal Parameters list before choosing an item from the top or bottom.	___	___	___
10. I choose bread *or* beverage *or* dessert *or* alcohol—one of four, or none.	___	___	___
11. I drink 8 to 10 (or more) glasses of plain water daily.	___	___	___

	More Often Than Not	Try to Make It Happen	Seldom or Never Accomplished
12. I choose hot cereal, cold cereal, or egg for breakfast.	——	——	——
13. When I'm not having protein at lunch or dinner, I choose a soup, All-Vegetable, or egg meal.	——	——	——
14. I eat a wide variety of vegetables.	——	——	——
15. If not hungry and thinking of food, I use repatterning techniques until the moment passes.	——	——	——
16. No matter how difficult it is to accomplish some assign-ments, I go back on The Pro-gram at the very next meal.	——	——	——
17. I monitor the frequency of Fillers in my log.	——	——	——
18. I skip a day or scatter at differ-ent meals the Fillers I choose.	——	——	——
19. I leave over one bite of food each day—one bite each meal, if possible.	——	——	——
20. I breathe deeply and stretch to relieve tension and stress rather than using food for this purpose.	——	——	——
21. Breakfast consists of one item, occasionally two.	——	——	——
22. Lunch consists of one or two items, occasionally three.	——	——	——

	More Often Than Not	Try to Make It Happen	Seldom or Never Accomplished
23. Dinner consists of one or two or three items, occasionally four.	—	—	—
24. I consume five or six items daily (with an occasional four-item or seven-item day), with one, two, three, or four items at dinner; one, two, or three at lunch; and one or two at breakfast.	—	—	—
25. I've been ordering, buying, preparing, and eating less food.	—	—	—
26. I regularly leave food on my plate.	—	—	—
27. I choose more chicken, fish, and veal.	—	—	—
28. I choose less High-End Protein, which includes cheese.	—	—	—
29. I have more energy and incorporate as much physical activity into my life as possible.	—	—	—
30. Every food choice I make reflects my ultimate weight-loss goal.	—	—	—
31. I'm feeding a smaller person.	—	—	—
32. The portion size of most items has been diminished by a bite, a slice, a sliver, a sip, and a swallow.	—	—	—
33. I am clothing a smaller person.	—	—	—

	More Often Than Not	Try to Make It Happen	Seldom or Never Accomplished
34. I think of myself as a smaller person and throw out big clothes.	___	___	___
35. I am buying smaller eggs, chickens, fruits, and vegetables.	___	___	___
36. I meet nutritional needs before choosing foods from the top or the bottom of the Meal Parameters list.	___	___	___
37. I applaud my triumphs and Quantum Leaps rather than beat myself up for things I could not accomplish.	___	___	___

38. What assignments are comfortable parts of your eating behavior?

_____

_____

_____

39. Enter an example of a physical, mental, and refreshing repatterning technique you use on a regular basis that is helpful to you.

Physical: _____

Mental: _____

Refreshing: _____

40. Name the most important Quantum Leap you have achieved.

Physical: _____

Mental: _____

Refreshing: _____

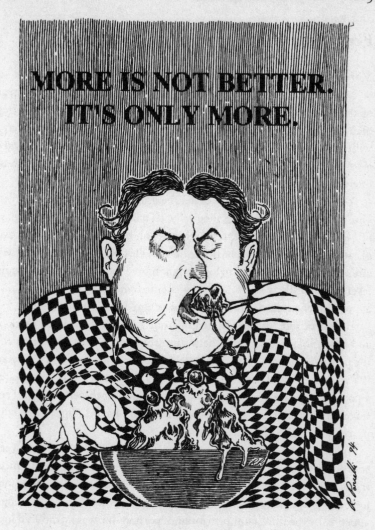

41. What assignments are not yet comfortable and what can you do to correct this situation? (Be specific.) Enter on your Needs Work page.

_____

_____

_____

42. Rewrite these assignments into your logbook for daily review.

Feed the Smaller Person You've Become

More is not better. It's only more.

Many people who try to lose weight are successful in many other areas of their lives. They are often perfectionists and high achievers. They make up their minds to do something and then do it. They often have willpower, responsibility, and the ability to delay gratification. *If I take these steps,* they think, *I'll get the result I want.* Yet they cannot seem to lose weight and keep it off.

Years ago, there was a diet called the grapefruit and buttermilk diet. One woman I knew thought, illogically, "If half a grapefruit and one glass of buttermilk is supposed to be effective, an entire grapefruit and two glasses of buttermilk must be better." So she ate double the recommended amount and fully expected to lose weight more rapidly. Although at some level she most likely knew better, she seemed sincerely confused and disappointed when she didn't succeed in reaching her weight-loss goal.

If four people, varying in height from 5'3" to 6'2", ordered chicken and broccoli in a restaurant, the waiter would not adjust each order for the person's height or body type by saying in the kitchen that one woman is 5'3", one 5'8", and the men are 6'0" and 6'2". Since a restaurant creates a portion based only on what it wants to charge, each person would receive the identical amount of food and would have to figure out how much of the meal he or she needed.

When I was losing weight, I realized the portions of many foods were enormous. Chinese restaurants, in particular, often serve a person a meal that could feed a family of four. In the grocery store, I see oranges that look like grapefruits and bananas that could have satisfied King Kong's appetite. By the time a uniform 4-ounce portion size was introduced into my life, I was so used to the big, bigger, and biggest of everything that I'd look at the smaller size and think that it looked so . . . small.

Strangely, though, when the meal was over, I always realized that my eyes had indeed been bigger than my stomach, because the amount I'd considered small was really enough. Elaine Boosler, the comedienne, still makes me laugh when she holds up an imaginary pint of ice cream and exclaims incredulously: "Serves four!?"

As you become smaller, your stomach shrinks. You fill up sooner. What has always been physiologically enough eventually becomes emotionally enough too.

When I have soup in a local coffee shop and am served by one of the thin waitresses, she puts one package containing two saltine crackers on the plate with the soup. The 250-pound 6' tall waiter gives me several packages of crackers. Both meals might be considered soup and crackers—two items. But in reality, one of the meals is really soup and crackers, crackers, crackers—three or even four items. The question isn't, How big is a portion size? The question is, How much is enough?

Many people are satisfied at lunchtime eating a two-item meal during the week, whether at home, in a restaurant, or at the office. But they might feel compelled to eat double or even triple that amount of food on weekends, or when they have alcohol. The amount of food increases even more depending on the number of people in attendance. Because the number of items, as well as the portion size, varies greatly from place to place and situation to situation, even a person who is most determined to lose weight remains confused.

A few years ago, Oprah Winfrey used a liquid protein drink to lose weight. She was so proud she had lost 60 pounds that on the day of her body's unveiling on her television show, she pulled a red wagon full of 60 pounds of animal fat onto the stage. The presentation was so dramatic that few of us who saw it will ever forget it. As she proudly showed off her new svelte figure she joked with the audience that she and her boyfriend "could now go to Hawaii and sit around the pool and eat bacon-avocado cheeseburgers."

She had successfully avoided food for six months, but she had not learned to feed the smaller person she had become. The rest is history. She gained the weight back.

The second time she lost weight, she learned a little bit more. But like many other people using food inappropriately, she was only okay when in a controlled situation or when her personal chef prepared her meals. From everything I've heard her say on her TV show, she does not appear to have learned to stop her habit of eating when circumstance ("We're in the neighborhood so infrequently . . ."), situation ("How often is it my fortieth birthday?"), or emotion ("I'm so happy" or "sad" or whatever . . .) comes into play. Is your every food encounter an exception to the rule, so that you end up with lots of exceptions and no discernible rule? These situations and how we respond with food are part of the ritual of food addiction. Do you see yourself eating for any or all of these reasons yourself?

You might be among the many weight control searchers looking for magic. *I'll reach my weight-loss goal but will continue eating the same foods, in the same quantity, and with the same ferocity, only I'll be the one person in the world who'll be able to keep it off.* That hasn't worked.

Most people who lose weight gain it back.

As you lose weight and continue to buy a little less, order a little less, prepare, serve, and eat a little less, you'll be a little less.

As you become smaller and begin to unravel the behavioral aspects of your ritual, you'll feel calmer because now you understand the mechanics of the ritual of your food addiction. Then you'll keep it off.

Mistaking Hunger

You are not hungry most of the time. You are not always hungry when something smells good, looks good, or tastes good, whether or not you think you are. All food is prepared to tempt your taste buds, even though you're not hungry.

You are also not hungry because there is stress, a deadline, pressure, a personal or business problem, anxiety, tension, it'smorningafternoon eveningwhenalonewithfriendsweekdaysweekendsdaytimenighttime moneyproblemsitraineditdidn'tcamewiththedinneritwasthere. You are not hungry 24 hours a day, though you might think you are.

There are many daily food encounters: friends offering food, a maitre d' describing desserts, and the smell of popcorn in a movie theater, to name but a few. Acknowledging the visual and emotional blitz helps interrupt the knee-jerk reaction that causes you to eat even though you're not hungry. Just knowing you are not hungry most of the time is a helpful piece of information.

You may even have pinpointed the reasons you're thinking of food—reasons that seem to justify your eating when you're not hungry. I've heard excuses as varied as "I got so angry because I couldn't get a cab" to "I got caught in a downpour without an umbrella." Many of these reasons might seem a valid enough reason to make you eat. They are not.

Certainly anger might tempt you to use food as a drug to keep the feelings down. If you eat when you're angry, does the anger go away? Or perhaps frustration weakens your resolve. At which point is *your* threshold for discomfort seriously challenged? Bored? At exactly which point does a yawn become a yen? Tired? When does food become a replacement for sleep?

Does the emotional pain diminish when you eat? Is the celebration any better because you come home stuffed, bloated, and full of gas, uncomfortable, and with lowered self-esteem? Is it worth it?

Consider, if you will, that your past behavior has not worked. A clear vision of what you're trying to accomplish will. Most of all, you need a mind open to the *possibility of change.*

One man I almost taught was so afraid to change that he was locked into where he hung his coat, where I sat, and where he sat. He was terrified I was going to pull off his covers and yank away his security blanket of whatever food he was holding onto—whichever food he thought made him comfortable. He was so uncomfortable with even the thought of change that he would not tell me how much he weighed or what he wanted to weigh.

Of course, it's possible that some discomfort might occur while you're changing. The very act of weighing less than you did before is a change, and there is no change without change. But there are ways to lessen the discomfort of the journey from where you are to where you want to be—to offer options, suggestions, tactics, tips, tried and true assignments that work more and more as they are practiced. After all, you learned to use food to calm yourself down. *You can learn a new method,* a new automatic response.

Do you eat out of habit, not hunger? Identifying habits requires guidance, introspection, and patience, but most of all honesty. Once you acknowledge, "Yes, I do *that,*" you can decide you don't want to do *that* anymore and begin to do something else instead.

It is unrealistic and self-defeating to expect to go from habitual, compulsive, or addictive eating behavior to a calm, rational, in-control eating person by reading a few pages in a book, even this book. You can, however, alter automatic, learned responses by creating new and effective alternative behaviors that will result in permanent change. The new behavioral choices add up to a permanent weight loss but incrementally, not over night. It's worth repeating: Your original patterns evolved over a lifetime. Now you can consciously plan the person you want to be.

Food does not contain a narcotic. Food has only the power you gave it by doing the same thing with it each time you encountered it. Food has the power you vested in it as part of a ritual distraction with your mind, many times since childhood, when you might have learned how to cope with stressful situations by using food inappropriately. It might have worked then, but it's not working now. Now we need to find a new way that will work.

I'll show you what to do if you are not hungry but are tempted. There are many things you can do when food is offered, baked, cooked, prepared, and presented just for you. Learn how to handle the compelling urges at the office, in a restaurant, or at home. Learn that an umbrella-topped pushcart, wafting a familiar aroma, doesn't always mean you have to eat a hot dog.

Hunger demands to be fed. An urge passes. Know the difference? The next time you're at home and thinking of food, and you just ate a little while before, set a kitchen timer for 20 minutes and *distract yourself with some activity*. Sometimes I set the timer, get busy with some other project, and when the bell goes off, I not only forget I set the bell, I'm not even sure *why* I set it in the first place.

One woman recalled a walk she took one summer day. She spied a man eating an ice cream cone (a visual stimulus). She used the mental repatterning techniques she'd created to distract herself. She'd practiced and repeated the words, "Alert. Alert. Cross the street," which she did while laughing. She reassured herself that everything was going to be okay, and she prompted herself to calm her breathing. "Two minutes later, I'd found the most adorable sequined hat in a store window," she recounted. The moment clearly had passed.

The techniques were there in her memory bank because she had written the specifics of her plan, reviewed it daily to remind herself of the details, and envisioned it in her mind, so that when the ice cream cone appeared, her new automatic response—to say, "Alert. Alert. Cross the street, take a deep breath, and keep walking"—kicked in. It is a process everyone can learn. It begins in your mind.

If you do not eat something when you normally would have, you might be particularly motivated to reach your goal weight for an upcoming wedding, class reunion, or birthday celebration. If you use willpower, self-control, good intentions, and inner resolve, you'll find the results temporary. The next time the same circumstances or food appear, you may be a little less motivated or a little more angry, lonely, tired, or bored, and you'll probably eat the food, only to reinforce your old eating behavior, which is what caused you to gain weight in the first place. There is no good intention, self-control, inner resolve, or willpower sharp enough to cut through the layers and tentacles of your very practiced and polished ritualized eating habits—habits gone haywire. If you ever had good intention, self-control, willpower, or inner resolve, you would have used it 5, 10, 20, 30, or 50 pounds ago.

If, however, you begin to change your overreaction to food by doing something else, you might end up eating the object of your desire, but you'll most likely not put as much on your plate, you'll eat a little less, stop a little sooner, and eat it a little less intensely than if you had not attempted some repatterning techniques.

The first time you do it the new way, it might feel awkward and uncomfortable. It is different from what you've done in the past. But no matter how uncomfortable you feel at the beginning of creating a new habit, nothing is as uncomfortable as having to choose what to wear based on how much of your body it will cover. Nothing is as uncomfortable as selecting what to wear based on what fits on a particular day rather than what is appropriate for a particular occasion.

Positive thoughts beget positive results, and negative thoughts beget negative results *whether or not you believe the words as you speak them.* When you say things aloud, the words you speak have even more power. Things you envision, repeated positively, get positive results if they are said aloud and regularly. Consistency leads to success.

Conversely, if you are thinking and talking about the negative, about your real or imagined failures, you'll manifest more of the same.

From the first thing in the morning until the last thing at night, read, reread, and speak the list of things you're trying to accomplish. Post the list on the bathroom mirror, throw a copy in your wallet, or use a reduced version as a bookmark. Picture your success. Imagine your success. Strategically place duplicate cards in your desk drawers, in your attaché case, and on, in, or near anything else you come in contact with daily. Surround yourself with the list of things you're trying to accomplish, and read and imagine it daily or more often.

Keep a written checklist of all the things you did accomplish (see the Quantum Leaps chapter for examples), so you can do them again.

Maintain a positive *I can do it* mental attitude, and positive results happen. Avoid negative words about yourself, such as *bad* or *failure* or *I blew it.* They are just words and do not apply to anyone who continues to try. "It ain't over until it's over," Yogi Berra said. I believe that.

For best results, attempt many kinds of change in your life. If drinking water doesn't help by itself, perhaps the water and deep breathing will be helpful. Sometimes water, deep breathing, changing location, *and* calling a friend is what you need. *It is the action of taking an action—any action—that gets the result.* It almost doesn't matter which techniques you use to repattern. What is important is that you take a swift, purposeful, and immediate action. The quicker the action, the quicker the moment of anxiety passes.

It is possible that sometimes you might try every technique available and the moment is still difficult. It happens. But that doesn't mean you should stop trying. It just means your results have not quite accumulated enough to effect a noticeable change. It doesn't mean nothing is happening. It just might be too subtle for you to notice. Keep doing it anyway. It accumulates. Continue trying, and from each seemingly failed, imperfect attempt, the structure of the old, destructive habit will be eroded another little bit. You will be that much closer to success. All those teeny little bits add up to eventual success. If you strike the habit enough times, it will eventually shatter.

There is no instant success. There is no magic. There is only the ongoing process of placing one foot in front of the other until the journey moves forward. It is never finished. Just like life, it is a work in progress.

It took many episodes of reinforcing old behavior to create patterns as ingrained as the ones you are trying to change. It takes many steps of new behavior until you're hooked on the new way.

There are four areas of repatterning that are helpful: *mental, physical, verbal,* and *relaxing/refreshing.* Sometimes one technique works, sometimes another. Every food encounter is different from every other one. Everyone responds to each stimulus differently and responds to repatterning techniques in a different way too. A combination of several techniques may be just the ticket when one is not enough. Be creative.

Identify your eating patterns. Even the seemingly insignificant ones, such as *it's only broccoli,* or *I only drink black coffee* add up. Do you mean an orange has the same significance as a piece of candy? What ritual thinking is in your subconscious? Are leftovers a problem? Does food preparation end up being one for you and one for the pot? Does someone else serve you your food at home, in the office, in a restaurant? Do you finish everything served to you?

One woman I teach had the habit of *eating after eating.* She battled that habit for many months. When I spoke to her last week, however, she reported a two-week period when she did not once eat after dinner. This lifelong pattern had finally been laid to rest. She is fifty-nine years old.

If you buy, prepare, serve, and accept a little less food, you'll eat less. Ultimately, you'll be a little less.

If you don't bring it into the house, you won't eat it. Out of sight, out of mind.

If it doesn't taste good or look good or satisfy the eye and palate, don't eat it. We all belong to a nation of people who finish everything on their plate. That is not necessary. *You may leave food over.* It's okay. Food is wasted if you put it into a body that doesn't need it. Better to throw it away. If you order less the next time, there will be less to waste.

When you go off The Program because you're human, you didn't blow it, weren't bad, or a failure. Don't beat yourself up. Simply get back on The Program at the very next meal. Try to figure out what you could do next time the same thing inevitably happens. The quicker you're back on your program, the more you'll want to stay on your program. It is becoming comfortable, enjoyable, and preferred behavior. Just being aware of your old behavior patterns enables you to choose new ones. Being aware is an example of mental repatterning.

Usually, water (a refreshing technique) and deep breathing (a relaxing technique) are enough to distract your attention until an anxious moment passes.

Think of things you can do if you're thinking about eating but know you're not hungry.

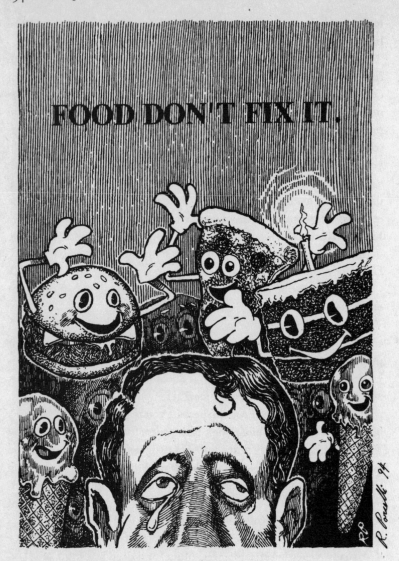

FOOD DON'T FIX IT.

Reasons for Repatterning

If you're thinking of eating and you've recently completed a meal, or if you are mid-meal and are most likely not hungry anymore, your goal is to change your thinking from the old destructive mode to a mode more likely to help you reach your weight-loss goal.

If you continue reinforcing your old behavior or only try to avoid the compulsion, chances are the attempt will be only temporary. But, if you change your old behavior to new behavior by repatterning, the difficult moment will pass, and the new behavior will eventually become the comfortable behavior. In order for this to happen, however, you must be consistent in your attempts. Consistency leads to success.

Following are action steps to take instead of eating. (The suggestions have been effectively used by many. Add two repatterning techniques that work for you in each category.) If you envision yourself doing each of these things and practice each action, it will become more comfortable. Say aloud and repeat the words *I can* before each phrase:

> *Physical*—I can move, change location, throw food away, go for a walk, clean a closet, exercise, call a friend, go to a movie, brush my teeth, drink water, read my affirmations, walk a dog, cross the street, take a deep breath, do head rolls, stretch my shoulders, stretch my legs, change activities, take a break, go to the rest room, take a nap, go to sleep early, leave the site of my anxiety, leave the room, drink water, use a treadmill, pick up the phone, read, open the mail, tend the plants, play the piano.
>
> *Mental* (things you can say or think to yourself *before* or during a food encounter)—I can visualize success, imagine a more attractive me, think of the reasons I want to change, know that eating doesn't change the outcome of anything except my waistline and self-esteem, deal more directly with thoughts and feelings, anticipate and plan ahead in detail the foods I am going to eat, anticipate and plan ahead the repatterning techniques I plan to use, imagine constructive ways to utilize my time, plan to succeed, recommit to my goal, visualize a smaller me, feel more comfortable with myself.
>
> *Mental* (things you can say to yourself *after* a food encounter)—I can say the moment has passed. I'm feeling fine. I won't remember the discomfort in a few minutes. I don't

Reasons for Repatterning Form

Note five or more repatterning techniques in each category that work (or could work) for you. For best results, use a combination of mental, physical, verbal, and refreshing techniques.

Physical (movement)

_____

_____

_____

Mental (things you say to yourself, e.g., I want to weigh _____)

_____

_____

_____

Verbal (things you say to others)

_____

_____

_____

Relaxing/Refreshing (food-free pampering)

_____

_____

_____

really want to eat. I'm not hungry. I'm okay. I feel great. I don't need to be drugged. I really want to be thin. I don't need to eat to make myself happy. I can say *no, thank you* to others as well as to myself. I really want to be successful and reach my weight-loss goal.

Verbal (things you say to others before or during a food encounter)—No thanks—I'm not hungry. I'm fine. I've had enough. I'm good. Nothing for me, but you go ahead.

Relaxing/Refreshing—I can take a deep cleansing breath, change location, take a stretch break, freshen my mouth, take a nap, take a bubble bath, take a hot shower, go to bed early, sleep late, have a massage, have a manicure or pedicure, pamper myself, read a book, listen to music, sit quietly, plan tomorrow's eating, review my affirmations, get tickets for a concert, go for a leisurely walk without money, slow down, complete a jigsaw puzzle, practice needlepoint, write a letter, go for a drive, go to a movie, rent a movie, put on hand cream.

Difficult moments will pass whether you eat or drink or not. Using any repatterning technique or combination of techniques will help the moments pass more comfortably.

A Trade-Off

When my awareness of what I was eating and how I was behaving was at its height, I realized I was buying, and eating, numerous candy bars, bags of potato chips, boxes of cookies, and pints of ice cream. Some days I bought only one of these items to eat. Some days I bought all of these items.

In my quest to create new, more constructive automatic responses to replace my old destructive automatic responses of "I see it I eat it," I wrote assignments for myself. I'd aim for one no-_____ day. This could be for my coffee and bagel habit, or my candy bar habit, or my must-have-popcorn-in-the-movie habit.

At the beginning, I chose one no-candy day, but the *compulsion to purchase* was powerful. When I was in my addiction and drifting un-

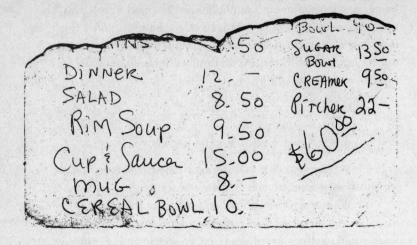

consciously into one of the stores where I was in the habit of buying candy, I'd buy tissues.

I'd buy those little fifty-cent packages of tissues, about the same price as a candy bar at the time. I'd toss the tissues into an unused drawer in my home. The new ritual took hold. In a few weeks, those little seemingly inconsequential purchases of tissues became a drawerful!

Had those few hundred packages of tissues been candy, cookies, or ice cream, there would be no memory of my having bought and eaten these items when I wasn't hungry—except on my waist, where it might have been ignored.

You can't ignore a drawerful of tissues. It is undeniable, visible, incontrovertible evidence of a *habit gone haywire.*

I then began putting, on a shelf in my kitchen, the exact amount of money I would have spent had I purchased each item—$1.79 for a bag of potato chips, $2.99 for a pint of ice cream, and so on. The money piled up even more rapidly than the tissues.

Some days I would have spent $10 and even $20. My assignment: Successfully transform an urge to buy something (a compulsion to purchase) into a no-purchase day. If I achieved this assignment, I could take the money I would have spent on these items and put it on a shelf in my kitchen.

Ordering Chinese food to be delivered would count if I had food in my home but wanted more or what I perceived to be better food. It was certainly faster food. In midtown Manhattan where I live, fresh, hot, and incredibly delicious made-to-order food can arrive in under 10 minutes—much more instant than if I were to shop, mince, slice, chop, and cook myself.

At the beginning, I didn't know what I was going to spend the money on. Then I saw some beautiful hand-painted dishes in a store window. I scribbled the price of each item on a 3-by-5 card I had in my bag. Every time I accumulated some money on the shelf in the kitchen, I'd buy a few dishes or a cup and saucer or a sugar bowl. I lost 50 pounds and still have a beautiful service for twelve. That's repatterning!

I still eat cookies, candy, and ice cream, but the portion is smaller than it was. I am smaller. More important, I don't desire these items as frequently as before either. Skipping, scattering, and variety help that. And it's fine. It's better than fine. It's enough.

And when I choose dessert or bread as part of a meal, I enjoy it even more when I place the food on one of these lovely plates. It's truly icing on the cake.

Repatterning by Anticipating and Planning Ahead

Any change begins in the mind. Imagine where you're going each day so you can plot a successful outcome to each food encounter. Imagine what food will be available or where you will get the foods planned for in each day's Meal Plan. Think about all the pitfalls into which you might fall. If you can first change the outcome in your mind, you can change the outcome of your meal.

The further in advance you anticipate the eating hurdles, the more easily you'll be able to create a plan of action to circumvent them.

When in a restaurant, do some verbal repatterning by asking the waiter questions: "With what does this food offering come?" This enables you to get exactly what you want, not what someone else thinks you should have. And if you know what you want before you enter the restaurant, you'll be that much closer to a successful outcome.

If you're alone, think about what you want for dinner. If you're going to be with others, tell them what you'd like to eat, whether they are cooking or making reservations. You might not always get your way, but if you never ask, you never will.

Whether you're traveling for business or pleasure, the best plan: Bring your own food. Sliced turkey travels well. See if you have it in the refrigerator or if you have to purchase it before you leave for the airport. I also travel with individual cans of tuna and small plastic bags containing shredded wheat or Grapenuts. Since milk is most likely not available, I eat with sips of the water I always have on hand.

Traveling at 2:00 A.M.? If you're not hungry and are going to pull the blanket over your head and sleep until touchdown, tell the flight attendant not to waken you if food is being offered.

If you're on a plane, however, you know that something edible is going to come down that aisle. Decide in advance what you are going to do with it. Decide you want to weigh _____ pounds.

Does the coffee wagon bell ring at 10:00 A.M. and 3:00 P.M. in your office, even though you don't work in an office anymore? Perhaps you're at home and avoiding work by using food as a procrastination device. Plan to head for the bathroom instead of the kitchen and brush your teeth, comb your hair, freshen your makeup, or splash on aftershave as a pick-me-up. If you're not at home, keep extra toothpaste in your attaché case, office drawer, or purse to swish around your mouth as a freshener.

When the smell of coffee brewing seems more than you can bear, aim for the water fountain. Don L. now keeps the electric coffee pot in his office filled with hot water.

Popcorn in the movies is similar to the coffee wagon. The movie does begin, you know, whether you have the candy or soda or popcorn or not. Bring bottled water to the theater. You eat only when you are hungry enough to commit to a meal—you who want to weigh _____ pounds.

You may be used to having after-work drinks with your coworkers or with your mate when you get home, but there are other things to do. Invite your coworkers to go for a walk (a physical repatterning technique) or suggest a visit to a museum that's open late at least one night each week. Pick a new favorite thing to do at least ten blocks away, and walk there and back (a physical technique); that's a mile or more in most towns. Use your imagination (a mental technique) to figure out what you can do at home with your loved ones that requires no food or alcohol. You'll come up with some enjoyable food-free fun to fill up your time and your life instead of your belly. Tell your friends you want to be with them, but you're just not hungry (a verbal technique) and only want some water.

Libraries provide great distractions. They do not allow food and are good places to browse for hours without once being reminded of food. If you find yourself in the cookbook section, however, change location. The idea is to distract yourself with activities other than food. To occupy your hands, try needlepoint, the piano, or a jigsaw puzzle. To occupy your mouth, try singing, speaking, brushing your teeth, or playing the harmonica rather than eating. Instead of extra food, get food-free tools into your home. What works for *you*?

If you arrive home at 5:00 or 7:00 or 9:00 P.M. and you walk directly into the kitchen to the refrigerator and begin eating, you're not alone. These behaviors are all conditioned responses. Know that the habit is changeable. The first step is identifying its existence. I used to find myself in my kitchen in front of the open refrigerator with my coat still on! I now close my kitchen door before I leave my apartment in the morning just so I am not in as much risk when I return in the evening.

You need some transition time between arriving home and having dinner. Unwind from the fast pace of the workaday world to the slower, more civilized pace of evening. No matter what time you arrive home, get out of your work clothes so you won't connect the clothes to the stress and tension you might be feeling during the day. Change into something more comfortable. Slowly, luxuriously, brush your teeth, freshen your mouth, stretch, and unwind. Read your mail; put on relaxing music; do a slow head-to-toe stretch. Practice deep breathing and slow exhalation techniques. Envision a thinner you. Put your feet up for a few minutes, and relax. The entire procedure might take 20 minutes, during which time your children and significant other should be put on hold. Tell them this is *your* time. Anticipate your usual after-work schedule and envision a better schedule you think will work for you. What if it doesn't? Keep polishing the new rituals. Remember: What you've been doing is not working. It's worth trying to find some new evening activities that don't revolve around your kitchen or food.

If you use food as a distraction from anger, frustration, and tension, think about the many things you can do to distract yourself from food.

Anticipate and plan ahead things to do when you're home for an evening. Get a sense of completion by cleaning a closet, ironing a shirt, washing a dish, practicing the piano, painting a picture, reading a book, going for a walk, taking a bubble bath.

Make a list of physical, mental, verbal, and refreshing activities you can draw on should the need arise. The list should contain easy as well as complicated things. They should vary in length and contain 2-minute, 5-minute, 10-minute, and 30-minute distractions, and some should last an entire evening. Reading your program notes is helpful.

During stressful moments, think about some mental repatterning techniques to use, such as imagining a thinner you and reminding yourself you want to weigh _____ pounds. Take a deep breath and distract yourself by referring to your Needs Work page instead of eating when you're not hungry. Enter every small, medium, and large chore you've been avoiding for months. In that way, if a magazine doesn't distract, maybe alphabetizing your Christmas card list will. You've been meaning to do that for years, haven't you? Find a hobby other than eating.

If you anticipate and plan ahead and are consistent in your use of these repatterning activities, the small steps become Quantum Leaps. What absorbs *your* mind and distracts you from food?

Repatterning by Thinking

Eating, or not eating, bread or dessert is clearly not the only issue. How many times a day or week do you choose black coffee, oversized salad, a half grapefruit? You hardly notice these foods. They are always a constant part of the landscape, like the china, linen, and salt and pepper shakers on the table.

Recent research indicates we receive information from all our senses; one part of the brain is used when reading, another part when writing, a third part when speaking, and yet another part when listening. Because you are exposed to more critical, negative images about yourself than positive ones, you must renew the information early and often as a reminder to think and act in a positive way.

If you don't keep a record of all the food you consume, the memory will be murky, and you will forget or deny small details. If you cannot remember it, you think you didn't eat it, and you further deny it has anything to do with your weight gain.

You might avoid taking an action that would let you know where you stand because no matter the outcome, you project that eventually you will have to do something about what you find out. You might have to change. You might further project that change is not as comfortable as not changing. It is actually the fear of something different that you resist. Yet your entire life is a series of things to conquer: tying a shoelace, buttoning a button, riding a bike, driving a car, learning to read, to type, and so on. It is the same with learning how to feed the smaller person you want to be. It is a process.

I cannot stress enough the importance of review. You've been fed a diet of misinformation, sometimes dangerous or unhealthy "have tos" about what not to eat and what to eat for such a long time that even though the outcome (how much you weigh) is far from satisfying, you continue repeating (in your mind) all those childhood bromides, such as *finish everything on your plate.* Some of the things you repeat in your mind have been added since you became an adult. Perhaps you've been encouraged to have a drink with friends because it's a celebration, or maybe you're being urged to order an appetizer or a drink because your companions are having one and they don't want to eat or drink alone.

You continue being a good child or good friend, following a yellow brick road of rules and regulations dispensed in childhood. Now you are a successful adult, maybe with children of your own. You support yourself and your lifestyle. Your old habits may be inappropriate for the responsible, reliable, successful, logical, clever person you are now. Yet you keep reinforcing your old habits just the same.

If, however, you review your assignments daily or more often, the new information becomes louder and stronger. Changing habits relies on *honest acknowledgment* of each problem and *relentless pursuit* of an appropriate solution.

There is resistance when it comes to change. Your old way is familiar and comfortable. You may not like the outcome, but there aren't many surprises. You resist letting go of the old and comfortable way. You block the very words you read. And you further deny that you are blocking and resisting. The beauty of daily line-by-line review is that even if you don't believe the words as you say them in your mind, eventually you do begin to change. Ultimately, the appropriate actions follow.

Since you don't know when you're ready to receive the words being read, it is important to review the narrative daily so that when you *are* ready, the correct information is right there for you to absorb into your routine. People who think they're doing everything the "right way" but are not getting the result they want realize after a couple of weeks that they are only scanning or glancing at each page. They imagine they know what it says. When I suggest they rewrite sections of the book if they inadvertently slip off The Program or need a push in the right direction to get back on The Program, they are surprised to find sentences and thoughts they think they've never seen before. A good habit to create is to envision everything as you read.

Envision a thinner you. *Dream* about the person you want to be. *Imagine* the way you'll walk and talk and look. *Picture* wearing the silk shirt you haven't worn since you bought it three years ago. *Think about* zipping up the slacks that stopped fitting the week you brought them home from the store. *Observe* the in-control you. How does he or she act? How does that thinner, more in-control you act around food? Feel good? Keep doing it.

Read your original thoughts about why you want to weigh what you want to weigh. Don't lose track of the reasons you're reading this book in the first place. Rereading the notes and pages you've highlighted provides a vivid reminder.

Anticipate and plan your entire day. Where are you going? When is food most appropriate? What foods are you looking for? Did you have a protein today? Do you need greens? Grains? Is the food on a plate? Is the Filler appropriate? Do you have a goal to consume fewer items at dinnertime? Are you achieving it? How are you doing with the 20-Minute Meal on your Needs Work page? Work on one or all of these suggestions and just keep reviewing; you'll incorporate things as you can.

Are you always thinking why you can't? Or creating *I can* affirmations? Meditation, motivational books, and audiotapes help face you in the right direction with positive thoughts offered by successful people. Focus on reaching your ideal weight. If other data distract you from your goal, keep pushing *you* into your consciousness by reviewing daily.

Think about the nourishment derived from each bite. Imagine the nutrients wending their way into your digestive tract, wandering into all the veins and capillaries, coursing through your bloodstream, being processed and utilized by your liver, kidneys, and other organs.

Learn how to eat the correct amount of food for a person the size you want to be.

A good way to retread old ways of thinking is to anticipate the old way a particular encounter would have gone if you hadn't given it any thought. Every time you realize there is a Possible Pitfall, change the outcome in your mind by thinking of an alternative food-free action you can take so you can continue your walk. Continue this process until you have successfully thought of a way to go one full day, from early in the morning until you go to sleep in the evening, choosing the foods in your plan and executing the repatterning techniques you plan on using. It is a challenge, but you'll have a nice sense of accomplishment and new feelings of hope. If your first attempt doesn't work, try again. Learn from the stumble. It took three months for me to conquer the 20-Minute Meal.

Whether you're creating success or failure, it all begins in your mind. Think about it.

I had two days of six items and feel so good about it.
As you suggested, I worked the schedule ahead of
time, in writing, with everything, including the Fillers.
It was a huge, huge help. (*Valerie D.*)

Repatterning by Moving

If you're not hungry but thinking of eating, take a physical action until the moment passes. In other words, move. It's a good idea to think about and write down the best possibilities so you won't have to do the thinking during a moment of anxiety. It can be a little motion or a broad physical exertion, but do it at the onset of discomfort, not after the discomfort has taken hold, which might cause you to spiral into a ritualized, overeating abyss. You want to aim for a swift, purposeful, and immediate action to help the moment pass.

If you've never done a leg lift in your life, I'm not the one to convince you to do one. Many people have bad backs, asthma, weak knees, recent surgery, and various other reasons they cannot do anything strenuous. I know a lot of others who have health club memberships, personal trainers, play golf or tennis regularly, and are still struggling with their weight. Still others cannot find the time. My conclusion (admittedly not based on anything scientific) is that physical activity is not necessarily a weight-loss aid. It is good for the head and good for the heart, and those are reasons to do it.

But unless you are religiously consistent with your physical activity, don't count on it for weight loss. If, for example, you begin your program weighing 200 pounds, when walking from the door of your home to a window in the living room, you'll burn X amount of calories. As you lose more and more weight, you'll have to walk from the door to the window and back just to use the same amount of calories as you did when you began. You might find it difficult to find the time to increase any formal workout to reflect your weight loss.

There are numerous physical activities you can do that can be incorporated into your day-to-day routine. Techniques that work for one person might not feel comfortable to another. Find something that feels comfortable to you.

- Move from a favorite place in which you are used to eating when you're not hungry to another one where you usually don't eat. You'll get used to the new place, and since it is a place where you normally don't eat, you won't feel the compulsion to do so. The new place is not part of your usual eating ritual.

- Keep moving until a difficult moment passes. Often I have to look at many magazines or writing projects until something absorbs my attention. I might move from my computer to the bathroom, to my bedroom, to the living room, and back to my computer, all the while searching for the perfect combination of repatterning techniques to help the moment pass. It always does.

- Rearrange your kitchen. Clean your cupboards, cabinets, and refrigerator. Get rid of the instant and always edible food. Everything in your larder should require preparation. Move foods to different shelves and to places you wouldn't expect to find them.

A tin-foil-covered half cantaloupe won't catch your eye on the bottom shelf behind a jar of pickles, but might not last an evening in a clear plastic wrap placed on the top shelf where you'll spot it immediately when you open the refrigerator door. You were looking for cold water anyway, weren't you?

- Take a walk without money, and see how many haunts where you might have bought something had money burned a hole in your pocket. If you don't buy it, you won't eat it. Buying is a habit too.

Late one rainy evening, I went for a walk in my neighborhood without money. The only store open was a greengrocer. As I mindlessly browsed among the instant prepared foods, the cashier asked if she could help me. I laughingly told her I had not brought money. I had purposely gone for a walk without money so I'd not be at risk.

"We know you," she smiled. "We'll give you credit."

Just what I needed: credit in a food store.

- Fill up on the architecture, the fresh air, your good feelings about doing something nice for yourself. Take a walking tour of your own city. Change other habits too.

George K. called, excited about breaking through his Maginot line of 220 pounds down from 250 pounds. "I already know what I'm doing on my ski trip!" he announced proudly. "I'm not only thinking about the skiing but the eating. I've never done that before," he admitted.

- When you do buy food for your home, divide it into individual portion sizes to freeze. If you know that one bowl of soup is enough in a restaurant but you consume the entire contents of a can when at home, repattern with the following steps:

    Prepare soup in a pot.

    Pour part of the soup into your awaiting bowl.

    Pour the leftover portion into an awaiting storage container.

Put soapy water in the pot.

Put the pot in the sink.

Freeze the part of the soup you're not going to eat.

Eat the part of the soup you're not going to freeze.

Enjoy.

Remember that in a restaurant, you'd never ask the maitre d' if there was another ladle of soup in the kitchen. You'd eat what ever was served, and that would be that.

Break down other eating rituals into small manageable, doable, achievable, proactive steps.

- Throw in the napkin! When all other techniques have been tried and you're still struggling to leave food on your plate, throw in the napkin. You've moved your plate, signaled the waitperson you've had enough, and the person on your left insists you have more turkey and stuffing. Desperate situations require desperate actions. It's Thanksgiving, and food has been prepared right up to the last minute. You may be feeling you'll never pass this way again, or that someone made something especially for you, or even "what the hell." If you've read your assignments and goals prior to entering the food pit and you have your eye firmly on the fact that you want to weigh _____ pounds, learn the napkin toss. When you're tempted to finish everything on your plate though you know you are not hungry anymore, pick up your napkin, dab your mouth, crumple the napkin, and throw it dead center in the middle of your plate. The napkin toss is especially helpful during the holidays and when there is gravy on the plate. This technique is not to be used often, but when it is necessary, it is very effective. Rarely, if ever, are you so in need of distraction or so bored that you resume eating from the same plate that contains a crumpled napkin soaked in gravy.

- Learn to say *no, thank you*. Learn to say *no, thank you* gracefully. If you are comfortable with saying no, others will leave you alone.

When loved ones insist they get you something from the kitchen every time *they* are bored, insist you'll be happy as a clam if they keep your water glass filled. Praise them each time they remember to do it and you'll have created a new habit that is helpful, constructive, and beneficial.

Mealtime Is Not Marathon Time

Mealtime is not a race to see how much food you can eat in the shortest period of time. Slow down, and savor each bite. Chew until the flavor is gone. Put your fork down between bites. Take a sip of water. Count to 20 before picking up your fork again. If with others, wait for the answer to a question you've asked.

The people with whom I eat often order more courses than I do. Eating more slowly than my friends and sipping a lot of water between bites keeps me as busy as they are but less food is entering my mouth. I don't need as much as they do. I order fewer items, eat more slowly, and pace myself to finish eating when they do. Perhaps I'm eating one bite of food and sipping several sips of water when they might be eating a bite of food for every sip of water I drink. No one notices, and no one cares. If I'm not hungry, I'm not hungry.

Enjoy the subtle differences in seasoning and preparation. Think about the nuance of the flavorings while you're killing time between bites. Fill up on the ambiance and fill up your life, but don't fill up your stomach. At meal's end, put your utensils on the plate, and push the plate slightly toward the middle of the table. Move your chair slightly away from the table. End the meal.

Walking

Incorporate physical activity into your day.

Do you walk to work and pass certain stores that proffer doughnuts, muffins, and bagels? Do these foods call your name? If you're already in the habit of walking, add another block each day until the territory being covered is done in the quickest possible time.

Walk briskly, and swing your arms.

Catch the man in the red hat; pass the lady pushing the baby carriage.

Pound the pavement. It increases your heart rate. Everyone can be passed, even the old jogger up ahead.

Reroute around stimuli by walking down a different street each day. If a candy kiosk blocks the main entrance to your office building, enter from a different door. Use the stairs before getting on the elevator, and reverse the process when exiting. (Of course, make sure it is safe as well as okay with the building management. Some stairway doors don't allow reentry on all floors.)

Keep moving. Find extra mileage by walking up escalators even though they are moving in the same direction you are. Dance to upbeat music. When washing dishes or ironing, march in place.

To add extra steps, park the car at the edge of the parking lot, and walk to and from the store. Unless it is raining, the spot farthest from the store is the best parking spot for you. Is your bank or cleaners conveniently located across the street or around the corner from your office or home? Unless it is a severe winter, find another branch a few blocks away, and walk there and back.

Get off subways or buses a block or two before your stop and walk to your destination. Enjoy the extra fresh air, and arrive more awake for work than you were before.

Buy an inexpensive pedometer. It is a wonderful addition to physical life and increases walking substantially. When you realize those miles can accumulate even around your home each day, you'll add walking to your daily schedule.

Walking broadens the horizons, clears the head, and thins your thighs. As you top your personal best each day, a wonderful bonus of increased self-esteem gets added to your list of accomplishments.

Create a walking course around, to, and from your office, home, and weekend getaway. Plan to walk a certain number of blocks each day, or a specific amount of time, such as 20 blocks or 30 minutes. Increase the number of blocks and minutes each day. Count every extra step as a victory. It's usually an occasion when you're not eating. It becomes a wonderful distraction.

Do everything you can to keep moving, but don't sign up for a lengthy health club membership or purchase exercise equipment yet. It's better to take a brief membership or even rent equipment. Many people have fully paid health club memberships they've never used. Unless you are totally committed to working out a specific number of times each week, rain or shine, you may be wasting your time and money. My exercycle became the most expensive clothes hanger ever purchased. When I finally sold it, there was a half-inch of dust on the seat and an eighth of a mile on the odometer. Of course, some people do own and use exercise equipment. Elaine P. purchases long movies, such as *Lawrence of Arabia,* and allows herself to watch the movie only during the time she is on the treadmill. The movies she chooses are very compelling, so she looks forward to getting on the treadmill in order to watch the next installment of the movie.

Stretching Is Physical Activity Too

Integrate extra stretches into your everyday life—a stretch here, an extra block walked over there. If you insist on being human and miss a few chances to walk, anything is better than nothing. Even a daily flight of stairs, up or down, is 365 flights at the end of the year. Look for stairs to walk. That becomes a habit too.

Working out, jogging, and running (even in place) are good aerobic workouts if you do them, and they tend to reinforce your new eating habits psychologically. Good intentions, however, don't usually fit in with many lifestyles, circumstances, or the fact that it is another late night at the office. Exercise only for pleasure. Then if you miss a day, a week, or even a few months, you won't feel guilty.

Reducing your food intake without increasing your physical output gives a positive benefit to be sure. The synergism of both efforts gives much more than the sum total of either.

Walk back and forth when talking on the telephone; stand when at your desk until it is necessary to sit. Disconnect the remote control from your television. The moments will pass whether you eat or not. Taking a physical action will help each moment pass more comfortably. Which physical activities would work for you? Make your very own list. Move.

Don't Panic Card

It is inappropriate to take your logbook to a wedding or cocktail party; *all* the information might be *too much* information. Sometimes a Don't Panic card is exactly what you need to combat the temptation to overeat.

Photocopy it and carry it in your pocket or purse and look at it discreetly when you're searching for your handkerchief. There are action steps you can do or think. They are designed to calm you down. If you prefer, jot your own ideas on a blank card.

Don't Panic Card		Conquer Your Food Addiction

1. Don't panic. Change location. Move.
2. Take a deep breath. Exhale slowly. Repeat, if necessary.
3. Calm down. Smile.
4. Think: Everything's going to be okay.
5. Think: I can do it.
6. Step away from the Twinkies. Change location.
7. Remember: You want to weigh _____ pounds.
8. Think: I'm okay.
9. The moment passed.
10. I'm feeling better than fine. I'm okay.

Repatterning by Relaxing and Refreshing

By now it's apparent that physical movement comes naturally and extra steps are doable and fun.

Most people seem able to accomplish thinking and moving. It is the technique of relaxing and refreshing that stumps even the most determined.

From early in the morning until late at night, you attempt to be productive, prolific, accomplished, organized and efficient. If you're walking, you WALK. If selling, you SELL. If cleaning, you CLEAN. If working, you WORK.

The alarm clock rings, you bolt out of bed, shower, shave, dress, eat breakfast, and the rest of the day is spent running from here to there, completing errands, keeping appointments, doing lunch, finishing projects. Once you arrive home, there is mail to open, calls to return, laundry to do, children to talk to, dinner to be prepared, dinner to be eaten, dinner to be cleaned up and put away, and whew! Not once during the day was there a relaxing moment just for you. Not once during the day were there a few minutes to watch the crowds of people race by as you soaked up some sun in the pocket park near your office or in your very own back yard. Very simply, you have not learned to relax and slow down, to take care of yourself.

Relax Yourself

- The most important thing you can learn to do is to breathe deeply (diaphragmatically), in through the nose, holding to the count of five, and exhaling through your mouth slowly while you count backward from ten to one. While doing this, relax yourself from head to toe: your hair, forehead, eyes, nose, cheeks, ears, lips, jaw, neck, shoulders, chest, and so on, until you've relaxed your toes. At the beginning, there may not be enough air for so lengthy an exhalation, but practice inhaling first, and then increase the distance traveled on each breath of air. This can be accomplished in a few days. It is a wonderful tool used for every manner of discomfort. I even do this on a street corner while waiting for a light to change.

- Stretch all over. Stand in place, even as you read this book, and slowly rotate your wrists, ankles (first to the left, then to the right), shoulders (first forward a few times, then backward), and head (side to side, forward then backward). Hold each position a few seconds. Luxuriate in the feeling of your muscles and tendons and skeletal structure. Get the kinks out. Stand in place, and then turn from side to side slowly. Just standing in place frees the lungs to fill up more easily.

Refresh Yourself

- Brush your teeth after each meal or when you suspect mouth freshening would be helpful. Carry toothpaste and a toothbrush in your purse or briefcase. If in certain circumstances, brushing is just not appropriate, a swish of toothpaste on a finger in your mouth might work.

- Splash after-shave lotion or cologne on your face. Put it in a plastic bottle with an atomizer spray. It is very refreshing and a nice late-morning or early-afternoon pick-me-up. If you have access to a refrigerator, aftershave in the summer is nice when cooled.

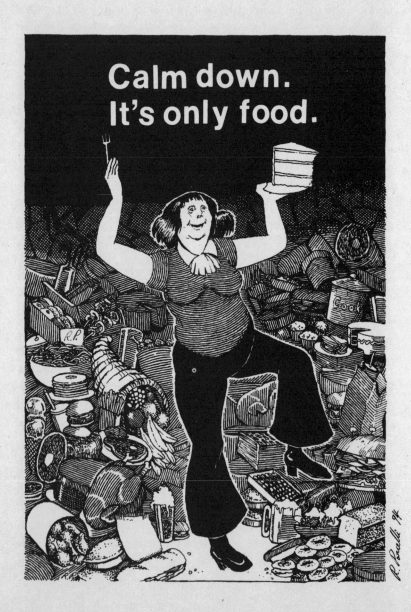

- Freshen your makeup by reapplying lipstick, refreshing your eye shadow, and dabbing cologne (cooled if possible) on your pulse points (behind the ears, on wrists, behind knees, and on ankles).

- If possible, floss.

If you are having lunch or dinner in a restaurant, take a moment and do these things in the rest room. Once you've freshened up after a meal, you most likely won't want to resume eating.

Slow Down

- Put your feet up and rest for twenty minutes. Force yourself to do this on a regular basis. Try it now.

- Go to bed earlier than usual two weekday nights a week, and get the same benefit as if you were sleeping late.

- Take a bubble bath. (You men can indulge yourself, too). And get an in-house massage. Wrap yourself in an oversized towel. Have all evening chores attended to before the masseuse arrives, and pay before you lie down. Then when the masseuse has tiptoed out of your home, you can drift into blissful sleep.

Pamper Yourself

- Give yourself a manicure or pedicure, or have a professional do it. If you ask, you'll most likely be able to get a mini-massage of the hands and feet, which feels great and is worth the price of the polish. When I get a haircut, the person who does the shampooing usually massages my scalp too. This is often more satisfying than the cut itself.

- Buy flowers instead of food, and festoon your home and office.

- Get tickets to a concert, and take a friend.

- Go to a museum.

- Browse in a bookstore.

- Surround yourself with soothing, relaxing music.

- Sit still and relax for a specific period of time each day.

- Read as a way of relaxing, but choose books you really want to read, not ones that are work related.

- Review your logbook. It is a good time to remind yourself of all your accomplishments. It will remind you of what might need additional attention.

And finally, learn to slow down, relax, and refresh yourself simply because it makes you feel good. Many people feel *guilty* about doing nice things for themselves, but *you are worth it*. When you feel good, everyone in your life benefits.

Repatterning by Talking

If you've recently completed a meal and are thinking of eating again, or if you're mid-meal and most likely no longer hungry, your goal is to change your thinking from a destructive mode to a mode more constructive that will help you reach your weight-loss goal.

Destructive thinking is, "It's so small, it couldn't possibly count," or "It tastes so good I cannot leave any of it on my plate," or "My clothes fit perfectly; I can afford to go off my program."

Constructive thinking is, "I know if I swallow it, it all adds up," or "It does taste good, but I'm not hungry anymore," or "My clothes fit perfectly, so I will continue doing my program."

In previous chapters, you've read about repatterning by thinking, moving, and relaxing/refreshing.

Thinking techniques (mental repatterning) include anything you say to yourself. You can anticipate and plan ahead before a food encounter, implement a litany of calming words and phrases to be thought during a difficult moment, and evaluate and adjust each food encounter, after the fact.

Moving activities include any kind of movement, whether minuscule or broad. You can move either you or move it (the food).

Relaxing/refreshing tactics are primarily used to reduce stress and make you feel better. Pampering yourself with bubble baths and massages are examples of things you can do for your body. No money? Trade those services with a friend. Soft music and light reading are examples of things you can do to relax.

The last piece of the equation is *verbal* repatterning—things you can say to others, that is, talking.

When it comes to overeating, you may not have learned to set boundaries for yourself, and if that is true, you may have a similar problem when interacting with others. It is important for you to find the correct *tone of refusal* so you do not spurn love or friendship.

First, learn to say three little words: No, thank you. Say it big: *No, thank you.* And again with conviction: NO, THANK YOU. And one more time: *NO, THANK YOU.* And one last time with feeling: **NO, THANK YOU!** You can vary this phrase with additional words—for example, "No, thank you, I'm fine." No, thank you, I've had enough." Or "It's wonderful, but I just can't eat one more bite."

You can also add a hand signal to the mix by extending your arm in front of you with palm down and fingers up while saying, "No, thank you." If you put your hand on your belly while slightly shaking your head no, few will doubt your sincerity. Of course, you have to convince others that you mean what you say (a win situation), or they will interpret your *no* to mean *coax me* (a no-win situation).

Watch your body language too. If you say no with your mouth but yes with your body by leaning toward the food you are refusing, your signals will be misinterpreted, and someone will tell the waiter or host to bring you a drink when you do not want one, or an extra spoon for a group dessert he or she has ordered.

Another effective phrase to practice is, "I'm not hungry" (although one woman's aunt asked: "What difference does that make?"). To the old you, the heavier you, it might not have made a difference. The new you, however, *never* eats without first being hungry.

Once you honestly know whether you're hungry, the next step is to get information by questioning others. Find out what your friends are planning to serve at the barbecue or dinner party to which you've been invited. Ask the waiter in a restaurant how a dish is prepared.

Tell companions what type of food you're looking for. Don't expect them to read your mind. If you really know you cannot find love among the guacamole, chips, dips, and salsa in a Mexican restaurant, open your mouth and tell your friends you'd rather go somewhere else. Express yourself clearly.

If you continue reinforcing your old behavior by always saying yes or just trying to avoid the compulsion to eat when you're not hungry, chances are that the attempt will be only temporary. But if you change your old behavior to new behavior by repatterning, the difficult moment will pass and the new behavior will eventually become the comfortable behavior. In order for this to happen, you must be *consistent* in your attempts. Consistency leads to success.

Victor Q. called from Florida to ask how he should handle a dessert-only party. I told him he should eat before he goes, get on the scale before he leaves for the party, recommit to his goal, and remember how unhappy he was only 20 pounds ago. When he arrives at the party, he plans to walk around with a glass of water. He'll visit with the 40 people he has not seen since last year. He's planning to behave in a way that is consistent with the way he conducted himself the previous week when he lost weight by eating only when hungry.

When I was at a similar party years ago, I listened to everyone else's comments about the desserts each person had brought; when asked, I white-lied about the ones I liked and didn't like, based on what I'd heard. There were so many people, so many rooms, and so many desserts, I am sure no one noticed whether I was eating. Meanwhile, I filled up on the fact that everyone was complimenting the thinner me they had not seen for a long time. This was a sweet enough pleasure for me. I brought pastry for the party, took home a piece of the dessert I wanted, and had it with my lunch the next day.

When it comes to food choices, open your mouth and convey your wish. Declare your desire, announce your aim, proclaim your plan, state your selection, tell your tactic, scream your strategy, divulge your design, trumpet your target, mention your intention, profess your purpose, say what you mean, whisper to your waiter, reveal your resolve, pick your preference, communicate, articulate, and exclaim your determination to get exactly what you want. In other words, talk!

Reviewing your notes before a party will remind you that you eat only when you are hungry enough to commit to a meal with food on a plate to be eaten with utensils, and you *never* eat foods from the top or bottom of the Meal Parameters list without choosing at least one item from the middle.

The first time I said *no, thank you* in a restaurant, the waiter actually walked away with a tray full of food. It was such a wonderful, powerful feeling—so powerful that I continue doing it to this day.

Which words and phrases could you use around food to get you exactly what you want? And while we're talking here, say: "I want to weigh _____ pounds."

Ten Things to Say to Refuse Food (But Not Spurn Love or Friendship)

Use the following or write your own list.

1. No, thank you.

2. I'm fine.

3. You go ahead and eat. I'll keep you company.

4. I'm not hungry.

5. I've had enough.

6. I'm enjoying just sitting here.

7. Nothing to eat but I'd love some water.

8. Not now; maybe later.

9. Thanks for asking, but no.

10. I just ate, *or* I'm going to eat [breakfast/lunch/dinner] in a few minutes.

And here are ten things you could instead think:

1. I just ate a few minutes ago.

2. I only eat when I'm hungry.

3. I'm enjoying the compliments.

4. My clothes are loose.

5. I feel great.

6. The moment will pass.

7. I wasn't thinking about food two minutes ago.

8. I'm enjoying the conversation and just sitting.

9. I'm fine.

10. I want to weigh _____ pounds.

Home Base

I'm writing this chapter a few days prior to the Fourth of July weekend when everyone seems worried about the eating situations they'll have to face: bountiful barbecues, delectable dinners, festive feasts, or potluck picnics, all designed to whet the weakest appetite and challenge your weight-loss determination. Perhaps a three-day summer holiday weekend is just another excuse to delay your weight-loss efforts until after Labor Day. Each holiday brings the ritual of enticing eating opportunities. These are the times when old habits take hold and pull you back, once again, to your previously practiced behavior. Your guard may be down because you've been on target with your eating program for weeks or months and you've forgotten you have old habits that may affect you seasonally rather than during your usual, non-celebratory, day-to-day routine. Just this past Memorial Day weekend, my friend Charles asked, "How could we be on the boardwalk in Long Beach, New York, without having the soft ice cream?"

These holidays come only once a year, and each one has an eating routine—a powerful food connection—all its own. From New Year's Day to New Year's Eve, if you've got a day, we've got a holiday (or event or celebration). And if you've got a holiday, we've got food.

Thanksgiving might have one set of food-related rituals (I'm smelling the turkey right now) that is different from those of Chanukah (latkes) or Easter (lamb, ham). Add to this list airplane travel, your birthday, anniversary, and a myriad of other celebrations with family, friends, and coworkers, each with its own food and eating tradition. If there are thirty-eight people in your office, there may be thirty-eight birthday lunches and thirty-eight birthday cakes.

When Beryl G. meets for dinner once a month with other day care moms, it always leads to eating and drinking overindulgences.

My friend Wendy has weekend guests at her upstate New York summer home where everyone cooks up a storm of specialties. Few of us could resist the toasted marshmallows she served for dessert one evening. If each one of these moments becomes an eating exception to the rule, you end up with too many exceptions and no rule.

When you are on target program-wise with breakfast, lunch, and dinner during your day-to-day nine-to-five lives, however that translates in your life, this is what I refer to as a *Home Base*. A Home Base is your home, office, or a restaurant (with or without people) where you comfortably achieve your mealtime goals. A Home Base is a safe harbor and can include people with whom you eat, foods you choose, and places in which you eat, all of which contribute to your weight-loss success.

My friend Lana and I eat together at least once a month. She is one of my home bases. If I suggest an All-Vegetable Meal, she says, "Fine." Sometimes we even share one dish. She's fine with that too. If I say I'm in the mood for soup, she says: "That sounds good. I'll have soup too." Chuck, however, is not my safest harbor.

When I tell Chuck I'm having soup, he says: "That sounds good," and adds, "And what do you want for an entrée? Do you want a drink? Shall we share an appetizer?" I can relax with Lana. I have to give a little more thought when ordering food with Chuck. I don't want to drift unconsciously toward a seemingly better-sounding or -looking dish than the one I planned on eating, which was fine just moments before I looked at a menu or heard Chuck's excitement at finding a favorite food.

A Home Base restaurant—the best are diners and coffee shops, which have a wide variety of choices available at any time of day—is also nice to have in your corner. A place near my office offers, in addition to its varied menu, baked potatoes ready for lunch, two kinds of homemade soup each day, eggs cooked to order, and hot cereal available until closing at 10:00 P.M. There are other shops where I can buy food by the pound, such as a quarter of a pound of sliced turkey, carrot salad, or coleslaw. Living in New York City, there are hundreds, perhaps thousands of restaurants where I am able to get exactly what I want 24 hours a day, seven days a week. With this type of selection available, it is easy to plan my eating and achieve my eating plan each day.

As soon as I leave New York City, however, the picture changes. Sometimes vegetables are prepared using a regional method I might not be used to, hot cereals are not always available, and I may not be accustomed to the local drinking water.

What you want to do is create a comfortable Home Base by practicing The Program *all* year; it is the repetition that makes the new thoughts and new actions comfortable and automatic. If you are eating hot cereal, cold cereal, or an egg for breakfast and have been losing weight or maintaining your goal weight, there is no reason to change your ritual just because you're not in your usual environment. If you order oatmeal or Wheatena or egg, you don't have to see the bacon and hash browns cleverly calligraphed on a menu. If you were home, you wouldn't look at a menu before deciding what to eat. You most likely wouldn't prepare home fries with your scrambled egg. Your goal is to take your weight-loss program with you and to *enlarge your* Home Base, so that no matter where you are in the world and no matter with whom, you are the same person with the same original weight-loss goal.

If you want to weigh your goal weight 365 days a year, not just when it's convenient, I recommend that you travel with a lightweight, extra-slim travel scale. If you pack the scale first, it will fit into your suitcase. If you pack it last, it won't.

"But I stay in the best hotels and they have a scale," you say, thinking, *This is crazy. This is going too far.* "Yes, they do," I answer. "But it is not *your* scale." Taking your scale on trips is taking your Home Base with you. You're taking along an important component of your weight-loss success.

The first trip I made after I'd lost my weight was to San Francisco for Thanksgiving. I didn't take my scale because my friends assured me they had one in their bathroom that I could use any time. This sounded fine in theory, but the reality was quite different.

My friends usually retire at 10:00 P.M. and read or watch television before they go to sleep. If I wanted to weigh myself in the evening, I'd have to do it prior to this time, undress, and redress. I'd have to repeat the process in the morning. When it got to be too much of a nuisance, I stopped doing it. On that five-day weekend, I gained 4 pounds.

When next I traveled in a recreational vehicle up the coast of California, I took my scale. My companion and I rendezvoused with other RV owner-friends. When my friend saw my scale on the bathroom floor,

Too Many Exceptions, Not Enough Rules

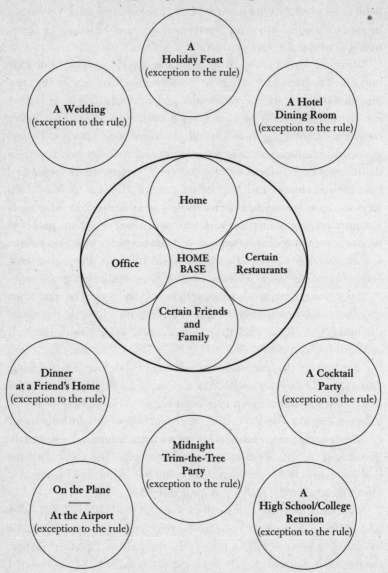

he thought it was unusual, and on the first night when everyone was gathered around picnic tables eating dinner under the stars in a beautiful national park, he mentioned that I had brought a scale. I feared people would think I was nuts. But in fact, the ensuing whispers were electric. "You have a scale?" "She brought a scale." "Which is your vehicle?" "Can I use it?" "What time do you get up?" The next morning, and each morning for the next few days, there was a line of all my new friends, male and female, outside our door wanting to use my scale. It is part of my Home Base, my safe harbor. If I know what I weigh each morning, then I know how to plan the rest of my eating day.

I recommend that participants of The Program do not discuss any of the details of it. Traveling with a scale might seem contrary to that suggestion. If anyone inquires, I tell them it is how I keep my girlish figure. We laugh, and they don't say another word.

Another aspect of my Home Base is to put food on a plate and eat with utensils. I attend numerous trade shows at the local convention center where the usual fare is hot dogs, hamburgers, and greasy sandwiches. Since I know this, and know it will probably not change, I bring my lunch, preparing it at home or picking it up on the way to the center. I do this for an airplane or car trip too. Usually, the only available foods are things I would prefer not to eat. I make sure to bring sufficient bottled water on every trip.

Keeping a Food Log, working with a Suggested Meal Plan, counting the Number of Items in a meal and in a day, or traveling with a scale might be part of your Home Base. These are things you can do anywhere in the world. Don't look for reasons to leave your weight-loss program at home when you're traveling. There will be plenty of situations when it is impossible to follow your plan exactly, but if you take along your Home Base, with more rule than exception, you'll be fine.

Dining Out

When you were in a restaurant as a child, did your parents admonish you to finish everything on your plate? When dining out, do you feel out of control with certain foods such as a basket of bread? Do you feel compelled to finish the entrée course you ordered even though, after you've eaten your appetizer, you're not hungry any more?

Restaurants have a strange influence over those who want to lose weight. Even the most determined eater starts to falter when faced with white tablecloths, tuxedo-clad waiters, and soft candlelight. The menu, which lovingly describes each item, presents a plethora of possibilities. Should you taste the truffles, decide on duckling, choose chicken Kiev, or savor the sushi? It is the indecision that tends to immobilize so many people.

We have touched on dining out earlier in the book, but now let's be more specific.

À la Carte Dining

As a general rule, there are certain rituals you can be sure you'll encounter when you're dining out.

Do you have a drink at the bar while waiting for your table? Does your hollow-legged companion order a bottle of wine and expect you to drink half? You might even be thinking, "What the hell," because once you start eating, you cannot stop. If it's ten o'clock at night and you're thinking about an appetizer *and* a main course, think again. It might be that the alcohol has once again clouded your mind and caused you to lose sight of your weight-loss goal.

The waiter brings a basket of garlic bread in an Italian restaurant, pita bread and humus in a Middle Eastern one, miniature loaves of black bread and sweet creamy butter in a steak restaurant. When the basket is empty, he brings more. You're most likely eating it because it's there.

If you're already physically distressed and the thought of even a few additional bites of food seems impossible, the meal is over. That, however, doesn't stop the waiter from describing appetizers, main course offerings, and desserts on the menu. You still haven't heard the laundry list of coffees, teas, and after-dinner drinks, when a plate of your favorite cookies arrives. You're most likely very tired at this point. Weight-loss resolve left about three hours ago. You reach out your hand, robot-like, and place a cookie in your mouth.

An à la carte encounter is but one of the *Dining Out* hurdles. There are more.

The prix fixe meal offers many more courses than you'd normally eat at home. The prix fixe meal gets you into the *it came with dinner, I paid for it I may as well eat it,* and *I blew it anyway* frame of mind. The prix fixe meal is usually a very good buy—but only if you would have ordered those very same courses anyway.

The early bird special is similar to a prix fixe meal, except that it's available earlier in the day.

Bread arrives on your table. It might be dry noodles in a Chinese restaurant, or tortilla chips in a Mexican restaurant. It's all the same: processed "prechewed" flour either buttered or deep-fried, and it comes with the meal, whether you ask for it or not.

All-you-can-eat restaurants offer unlimited quantities of wine, beer, salad, bread, entrée, and starch, all for one low price. Any number of salad toppings and dressings are attractively displayed, along with the specialty of the house, be it beef, chicken, ribs, or shrimp. Sometimes it is all four. There are so many foods from which to choose, it is hard to decide. You might fill your plate with a little bit of everything, making it necessary for two other people to help you carry your food to the table. Your companion invariably points out that you missed an especially special something, and you signal a waiter to bring you some of that too.

A drink with friends (in someone's home) doesn't seem like much. It's just a drink, and a beer or a martini does sound good; it's been a rough day. Maybe you think a drink is the only way to share a pleasant moment with people you like. Many of my friends serve something along with drinks, and although I do not eat before I eat, per the Meal Parameters list, no one notices when I don't, and even if they do, they don't care. If others want more than one drink, I just say, "Not for me, but you go ahead."

The other night after dinner, I invited a group of people back to my apartment for coffee, cake, and wine. I sipped hot water from my favorite cup. I assume my friends had a nice time even though I wasn't drinking alcohol or coffee or eating a piece of cake because they didn't leave my apartment until midnight.

The happy hour is an institution designed by bars and restaurants to bring in office workers before they head home. It is enticing. Many restaurants offer happy hour nibbles—chips and dips, nuts and pretzels, or more elaborate spreads. One New York City pub has an entire buffet of sliced beef, an entire roast turkey, salads, rolls, and all the trimmings free with the purchase of two drinks. Another offers cheese and crackers, miniature pizzas, chicken wings, and the like for the cost of a beer. A Mexican restaurant might have salsa and chips served by the basketful with every margarita. Everyone knows of at least one place like this.

If your companions want the bread on the table and it's not one of the choices you'd written in your plan, put it near them. *Then build a salt-and-pepper-shaker-flower-candle-water-glass* wall. If no one else wants bread, move it to an adjacent table, if possible, or have the waitperson remove the basket.

And who of us has not fallen into the trap of having one more drink because John is paying or it's Mary's birthday, or just to keep your friend company because he or she doesn't want to drink alone? Of course, if you succumb to the call of the cocktail, you just might forget that none of these circumstances is a reason to eat unless you're hungry. And you want to weigh _____ pounds.

Coffee shops and diners offer a wide variety of foods—a little something for everyone, from bagels, muffins, and all manner of bread, to eggs and omelets. The sandwich board includes double-deckers and even triple-deckers stuffed with pounds of meat served hot or cold. These restaurants also have many soup offerings, cold-cut platters, appetizers, side orders of potato salad, coleslaw and pickles, fruits, juices, beverages, and delicious desserts. My only comment about this type of dining-out encounter is, *be prepared.* Most portions are enormous, and I urge you to share. Some portions might serve two, three, or even four people. Don't assume half is yours.

I was once in the Carnegie Deli in New York City when a woman ordered matzo ball soup, which arrived containing dual matzo balls, each the size of a softball! The look on the face of the woman who had been served this gigantic-sized portion of soup was one of sheer amazement. We, at adjacent tables, were amazed too.

Pay-by-the-pound salad bars present a plethora of cold offerings and almost as many hot selections—truly a global smorgasbord. You can place as few as one olive and one peapod into your awaiting plastic container, or serve yourself heaping portions of macaroni and cheese, mashed potatoes, and chicken Kiev—all for the price of $4.99 or $5.99 a pound. Hot or cold, the chef making the salad bar offerings is knowledgeable to almost every palate. When I was heavier, I frequented salad bars and put a little of everything into my container still ruled by my Addict Pea Brain telling me *It's so small, it couldn't possibly count.* But it does count. So when you're faced with the challenge of a salad bar, think in terms of 4-ounce clumps.

Each 4 ounces is an item. If you go to a salad bar and know that you want two items and one of them needs to be a protein, it is simple. You could have one 4-ounce clump of tuna or shrimp or chicken salad. You might put a few shrimp with your tuna, but aggregately, the protein size will be about 4 ounces or less. Then even if you select a few sprouts, two olives, some shredded carrots, and some green vegetable, that clump of vegetables will be 4 ounces. When you check out at the register, the plastic container is weighed. On the left of the scale, it will tell you it weighs .25 (¼ of a pound, a 4-ounce clump, an item). If the scale reads .50, that is a half-pound of food, two items, and so on.

Street eating in an urban setting has become a literal global smorgasbord. It is all so portable. If you've got fingers, we've got Finger Foods— the ultimate dining-out experience.

Do you think that if food doesn't hit a plate, it doesn't hit a hip? That is the problem with vendor food. Because you walk with food, destroying the "evidence" as you go, you act as if it doesn't count. Bears repeating: *If you swallowed it, you ate it, and it all adds up.*

To help you make your way safely through the minefield of souvlaki, hot dog, and ice cream pushcarts, here are some hints:

- Make sure it's a meal. Others get in trouble because they have lunch *and* food from under the umbrella.

- Don't walk and eat. Every meal (including the shish kebob you buy on the street) needs to be eaten with utensils and should last a minimum of 20 minutes.

- Find a hospitable corner where people-watching can be as much fun as the food.

- If pushcart avoidance seems the best tactic for you, don't despair. Despite the hordes of vendors in certain parts of town, it is possible to steer clear of most of them if you pick your routes carefully. If one avenue is crawling with caterers, try an alternate street. If you take the same path every day, experiment until you find a route with fewer carts, fewer temptations with which to distract yourself, and different scenery.

I once exited from the north side of the Grand Central Terminal and the old Pan Am Building in New York City and bumped into a wall of a dozen carts lined up smartly on the street. The smells of grilled Italian sausage with onions, fried steak, and freshly baked chocolate chip cookies caught my olfactory senses like a deer in headlights. I fought like crazy to cross the street even though my senses had been sandbagged.

It may be hard not to succumb to the sight and smell of street food, but if you ask yourself if you were thinking of food or if you were hungry seconds before seeing the food, you'll be surprised how often you'll answer no and walk on by.

When I was growing up in Florida, where at that time there were no hot dog stands on the street, my father never thought of having a hot dog. I don't remember his ever eating one except occasionally on a plate with baked beans. Yet as soon as we arrived in New York City, the home of his youth, he'd pull the car over to a curb to order hot dogs with sauerkraut and mustard (the way he liked them) for all of us. His conditioned response from so many years before kicked in as soon as he saw the familiar umbrella. He did what he'd always done.

He was only in New York twice a year, so his occasional indulgence wasn't a problem for him or for any of us. I now live in New York and pass hot dog stands many times each day, but I don't act on it because I know it is merely a visual stimulus, and not a reason to eat. How many times a day do you act on a visual stimulus? How many times each week (month, year) do you act out a knee-jerk conditioned response?

Now you know some of the traps—they are plentiful. Can you anticipate them all? No. You can never anticipate every eating possibility, but you most likely have a pretty good idea of what is out there from experience. And you should have a clear vision of what you want to accomplish at each meal before you leave your home.

Think about some of the *gotta have it* rituals you've created in various food establishments. Do you always buy popcorn when you go to a movie? Do french fries always accompany your hamburger? Do you always eat the white rice that comes with your Chinese food? Think about some of the things you can do to change the outcome:

- Plan the content of each meal in advance, *in writing*. Work with your plan. If you know you are aiming for an All-Vegetable Meal, when someone suggests pizza, you'll be thinking of an onion/pepper/mushroom slice with a salad on the side.

- Be aware of the Number of Items you consume each day. By tallying the number of items you've already eaten that day, you'll know how many items are left.

- Be aware of *portion size*. Everything that is served to you will most likely be more than you serve yourself at home. There is no penalty for leaving food on your plate or on a serving platter. Think about sharing with a friend or taking home the leftovers for another meal, another day.

- Reduce the anxiety of leaving food on your plate by putting less on your plate to begin with. Remember that you're either trying to feed the smaller person you want to be, or you're feeding the smaller person you've become.

- Scatter your Filler choices. No matter how you try, you can't possibly taste it all at the same meal. You can, however, have a drink tonight, dessert tomorrow at lunch, bread at breakfast two days later, and maybe tea with dinner two days after that.

- You could vary your choices further. If in an Italian restaurant, choose pasta primavera as a main course one evening. Ask if there is a half-order, particularly if you're eating later than usual. Another evening you might order eggplant and mushrooms with sautéed spinach.

- The scattering technique is very helpful when dining out. Have a slice of garlic bread if the last time you had Italian food you didn't have it.

You pre-plan your day with regard to your clothing and your work. I heard there is going to be a rainstorm this afternoon. If I don't want to get wet, I plan to put an umbrella in my tote bag.

Make a plan, grab your resolve to at least try, and save yourself from gaining weight (or sabotaging your weight-loss plan) by anticipating the problems before each meal and thinking about the best solutions for each unique situation.

Hungry? Begin eating.

No longer hungry? Stop eating.

Now, take a deep breath. Difficult Dining Out moments pass whether you overeat or not.

The Weekend Guest

Consider this true story about being a guest:

> When I was heavy and friends invited me to Fire Island or the Hamptons for a weekend, I used to pray for rain. I was so embarrassed to possibly have to parade around in shorts and a skimpy top with my triceps flabbing in the breeze like a flag of skin, my thighs flopping up and down when I walked. Makeup dripping down my face, sweating like a pig, mopping my face with a wad of tissues, but still I won't take off my long-sleeved shirt.
>
> Wear a bathing suit? Totally out of the question. Cruel, heartless, thin men and women have all obviously designed them.
>
> My friends should only know. They spent tens of thousands of dollars to rent a summerhouse, and I prayed for rain. (*Raye E.*)

Jeff actually called Wednesday night from San Francisco to say he wanted to go to a popular New York deli for a pastrami sandwich as soon as he arrived Saturday night at 9:00 P.M. I was lucky. I had a few days to anticipate and plan.

Living in New York City, I entertain many friends from out of town.

They drop in when business brings them to the city, and they each have their favorite food haunts and must-haves: New York steaks, Jewish-style delicatessen, great Chinese food, and street vendor choices, such as hot dogs, salted pretzels with mustard, sausage and pepper heroes. They also purchase the proverbial bag or box of something to eat after dinner, before we go to sleep—sometimes even a slice of pizza. It's right across the street from my apartment. So convenient. So delicious. So portable. These friends readily admit they eat like this only because they're on vacation.

Ask your friends about their preferences so you can incorporate their favorite foods into the ones you're planning.

Anticipate your requirements and needs too. Then you can create a Meal Plan to accommodate you *and* your friends. No matter what your friend may want to order in a restaurant, most eateries offer a wide variety of food, and you'll be able to find your preferences too. Part of the fun of eating in a restaurant is that everyone can order exactly what he or she wants.

If you end up in a delicatessen, you can work that pastrami platter (a High-End Protein) into your plan, or if you're looking for a soup meal, choose pea, mushroom barley, or chicken soup with noodles or matzo balls. You can also introduce your friends to your favorite Indian restaurant for an All-Vegetable Meal.

Let friends know how delighted you are with your choices (verbal repatterning). Fill up on the fact that you're glad to see each other. Food is but one component of the visit.

Don't underestimate how certain people might trigger overeating episodes. One man told of a twenty-year vacation from the pizza-and-a-six-pack-of-beer-habit he'd perfected while studying for college finals, only to have the habit rear its ugly little head once again when a former college roommate visited him for a weekend.

Remember: Your friend's visit will not be enhanced one bit if you gain weight, only to dread the next encounter.

I spent a terrific snowy Thanksgiving weekend with a friend playing gin rummy one night and Scrabble the next. We took turns refilling our water glasses and putting logs on the crackling fire.

What could *you* do so a weekend guest won't interfere with your weight-loss success?

Weddings, Bar Mitzvahs, and Cocktail Parties

**Don't skip meals. Starving all day as an excuse to overeat
at a party doesn't work.**

What to Expect

A movable feast of elegant edibles, platters piled with a plethora of pip-
ing hot possibilities and crackling cold comestibles to be devoured with
flatware or fingers, scrumptious sweets for every tooth, plus spirits by
the shipload. Some celebrations lend themselves to predinner cocktails,
smorgasbord selections, an hors d'oeuvres hour, and then finally dinner.
Of course, there are after-dinner liqueurs, three varieties of coffee, six
kinds of soda, several special teas, and free-flowing alcohol. Most parties
generally have a wall-to-wall conveyor belt of food that just keeps rolling along.

There are varieties of cheese and crackers, chips and dips, breads and
spreads, and concoctions of condiments you haven't seen since the last
time you attended a similar soiree. All the attractively prepared foods
are lined up on tables like little soldiers waiting for your salute.

With the sounds of partying ringing in your head, you move through
the throng. Almost to prove to everyone else that you are a good guest
and enjoying yourself—or not watching your weight, which is forbidden at a food fest—you make sure you do taste it all. You maintain your
clean-plate-club membership and finish eating everything, though you
know you continue to eat even though you are not still hungry.

There are adorable dishes, bowls, plates, and platters with finger
food strewn everywhere. As you walk through a party, food leaps off the
tables and into your mouth. "I don't even remember eating it," Rose J.
mentions as she recalls this trance-like state after finding herself feeling
too full at the end of a party.

Some Things to Do

Remember you have a weight-loss goal. You're in charge. You want to
weigh _____ pounds. And these parties are not the Last Supper.

They are just another meal. Reviewing your program notes *before* a party is most helpful.

See which foods are available; you can usually find what you want among the excess.

No sandwiches for you (Finger Food, you know), though there is a wide variety of breads should someone else care to make a sandwich.

Don't underestimate the role your anxiety plays in determining your signals of hunger and satiation on these occasions. Anxiety is not a reason to overeat. Make sure you've allowed plenty of time to relax before you leave for the function. You might consider having a Fourth Meal of cereal before you leave your home.

When you write your plan, remember that alcohol causes lack of resolve and might compel you to drink even more alcohol and eat more food than you've planned. I know I said that before, but it's worth repeating. Be extra cautious when drinking at these functions, especially if you're suffering with social anxiety or fatigue. If you must drink, choose wine (or, if you prefer, beer) over hard liquor, and have it with your meal. Drink water in a wine goblet as you mingle with the other revelers. No one will know, and no one will care. When sitting at a table and eating, sip from your water glass before and after every sip of alcohol you take.

When someone else is preparing the food, overeating possibilities increase to the tenth power. The aroma. The beautiful presentation. Food choices are endless, and although culinary creativity is refreshing, *make sure your brain is in motion before you put the fork in your mouth.*

Plan ahead, in writing, as far in advance as possible. Think about what to eat before the smells, sights, and sounds seduce you. Ultimately, it's a numbers game. And the person consuming the fewest items at any meal wins every time.

Alert. Alert. Flying rumaki (bacon-wrapped chicken livers) arriving on a tray from the right. Are you having trouble tiptoeing through the turkey tetrazzini? It is helpful to remember, when eating any dinner meal, that you need only enough Food/Energy to take you from the hour you're eating up to bedtime. Have you tasted the shrimp puffs? To die for. Did an "oooh" and an "aahh" coming from someone's mouth turn your head toward a tempting taste treat rather than away from it? Keep moving, and remember how good you'll feel when you reach your goal weight and how unhappy you are when you overeat and gain weight.

Eat breakfast and lunch the day of the party so you won't use that as an excuse to overeat.

Plan, in writing, which categories of foods you're going to eat. Is it a protein meal or one with vegetables? Decide how many items you're going to consume. Is it a one-, two-, or three-item meal? Know which Filler you want more than another. Is dessert one of your choices? Don't taste all six; select a favorite, just as you'd do in a restaurant.

During the festivities, whether in your home or someone else's, speak to everyone. If it is a business function, it is easier to make your point or make a sale if your mouth isn't full of food. The objective is to find a focus other than food.

When at a party, walk, move, dance, change location, go to the rest room, stretch, mingle, relax, deep-breathe, and enjoy all aspects of the get-together. Food is just *one* of these.

The question isn't, Do you want the shrimp puff or the vegetable crudités? The question is, Are you hungry? Do you want to weigh your present weight next week or month or year? And how do you want to appear in the party picture, which will be around next week, month, year, and forever?

At someone else's party, food is just as abundant as at your own, but there may not be as many Program choices from which to choose—and perhaps none at all. It might be that all that is available are canapés and hors d'oeuvres, wine and fruit, coffee and cake—Finger Foods. If this is the case, think about having dinner before or after the party.

Years of practiced and perfected rituals come into play at a party, least of which is eating to please someone else. Yet I've heard many men and women say, "If I eat this [whatever *this* may be] I won't have room for that," and the host(ess) leaves them alone. Practice your tone of refusal so it's friendly and clear.

Your old diet mentality is to think you'll have the bare minimum—perhaps a piece of fruit and a couple of crackers. That thinking has not worked. You're reinforcing your behavior of eating when you're not hungry enough to put food on a plate, eating with utensils. If you make all parties an exception, you'll have no rule. The assignment is to be creative about following your plan so no one will know that you're doing anything special—to learn how to make your host(ess), as well as yourself, comfortable. Not every party is difficult. Most friends serve dinner at a reasonable hour. They are aware you might have to be up very early with young children or to go to work. And the content of food has greatly improved over the years too. But every now and then it is a challenge.

Wendy M. recounted a one-hour school meeting where everyone was gathered around an enormous pile of pastries while juggling a beverage and a conversation. For the first time she was mindful of the ritual and drank water, then left. Food is offered whether you are thin or not so thin.

Ultimately, do the very best that you can do under the circumstances. I'm at many functions where I hear others saying, "No thanks, I'm fine," and "None for me."

If you're going to someone else's party and you know for a fact they serve only hot dogs, hamburgers, and steaks at their barbecue, offer to bring some chicken, fish, or turkey franks, and a tossed salad for yourself and some other guests unless you've planned to have a High-End Protein on that day anyway.

During one Christmas, I, along with several hundred other people, was invited to a trim-the-tree party. Although the invitation said dinner, there was no apparent food in the kitchen and nary a caterer in sight at 9:00 P.M. I learned that it was the tradition of the hostess to serve wine and cheese all evening, then a complete pasta dinner at the stroke of midnight. Several of us were the hostess's new friends and had not eaten earlier as had the other revelers who'd been to the hostess's previous holiday parties. I tried to make do with some cherry tomatoes, a slice of cheese (from the middle of the Meal Parameters list), and one cracker (from the top of the list) which I broke into a dozen small bites. Was it the best choice? No. It was the *only* choice. I learned from that evening. I'm more thoughtful and prepared now.

It is a little trickier when the party is smaller. Anticipating and planning ahead helps.

If the bill of fare is buffet style, walk the distance without a plate. Select carefully in your mind. When you're sure the number of items and selections correspond with your original plan, then take a plate and put food on it. Serve yourself as if in a restaurant. Make choices based on what you've planned and the fact that you want to be at your ideal weight 365 days a year, especially when there are so many challenging choices on the china. Sit down with your plate. Eat slowly and thought-fully for at least 20 minutes while catching up on the news with family and friends—the reason for the party in the first place.

The party's over.

The kitchen is closed.

Thank you for coming.

Your Party

If it's your party, you'll most likely want to sample your tried-and-true recipes for deliciousness because you doubled or tripled the recipe for the event. Or perhaps you taste everything the caterer delivers to make sure the delicacies are as delectable as you thought they were when you selected them several weeks before. A missing bite of this and a taste of that won't be noticed, you think.

If munchies and nibbles are to be scattered throughout your home, place them on paths on which you're less likely to travel during the get-together. There are no munchie-food police should you decide not to serve pretzels, peanuts, popcorn, or potato chips. But whatever you serve, arrange the bounty on three-fourths of the coffee table. Sit near the corner where the candles and decorations have been arranged.

Before your guests arrive, make sure there are plenty of storage con-tainers available for leftovers. Make portions of food for another meal and freeze them.

If there are leftovers in the refrigerator, they will be picked at until all that is left is a memory, and eventually you'll forget that.

Not sure you can handle it? When in doubt, throw it out! This is no time to be in denial and believe you can handle a kitchen full of pre-pared, instantly available foods. You cannot. If throwing food away is difficult, give it to a neighbor, your doorman, or a homeless shelter, or send leftovers home with your guests.

If you've thought through the details of what you can do before, during, and after each party, from the time you set the date or accept an invita-tion, everything should go rather smoothly. There's always the possibility that a friend will walk in at the last minute with an unexpected key lime pie (my personal favorite). It's late, you're tired, and you're looking to distract yourself from the abundance of chores you need to work on before you go to sleep. You're tired, not hungry, but even if you pop something into your mouth, take heart. You most likely did better than if you had not given it any thought at all. You'll do even better the next time.

There is always one more party just around the corner. As a matter of fact, there's a wedding coming up, and you're invited.

A Wedding Reception

You and I are cordially invited to a wedding ceremony and reception.

A beautiful bride. A handsome groom. A lovely ceremony.

"I do."

"I do."

We arrive at the wedding reception with throngs of other celebrants and are ushered into an open bar area. White-gloved waiters roam the massive foyer carrying trays of champagne glasses and try to make eye contact with the thirsty. They traverse the travertine marble floors with enormous bottles of red and white wine, wishing to wet our whistles with their wares. The cacophony of music, laughter, glasses clinking, forks clanking, and shoes clicking on the marble floor add to the festive atmosphere. Gershwin fills the air. My escort and I dance in the semi-darkness, imagining ourselves to be Fred and Ginger, with others eventually joining in for a conga line around the front door.

When we move up the stairs out of the entranceway, no sooner do we dodge the dim sum than a tray of puff pastries is presented under our noses. We arrive at "food central" on the second floor and almost bump into a table the size of a football field laden from goalpost to goalpost with offerings of shrimp, and canapés of meats, and cheese. The buffet table is straining from the pounds of produce overflowing the boundaries of each platter and bowl. And all around us are hors d'oeuvres hovering, canapés calling, and bonbons beckoning.

I overhear a discussion about the dinner to come: "Do you mean we've been eating and drinking for an hour and now we're going to eat again?" a woman asks her companion. "Yes," he answers, as he consumes a caviar-covered cracker.

The wedding reception is nondenominational, but it could be any ethnicity. Each has its own set of ritual, pomp, and abundance.

We breeze through a buffet table of seductive smells and tantalizing taste traps. Our eyes dart from food to decorations to the bejeweled women on the arms of tuxedo-clad men. Sensory overload. We smile for the camera and pose for perpetuity.

We join a group of old friends and catch up on the news. We sip water from wine goblets provided by the bartender. We're all dressed up, there is little else to do other than eat, and we don't want to be left out or impolite. The reason we're here in the first place is to celebrate an event, not focus on food.

Things You Can Do

Eating breakfast and lunch is vital. You're going to be dancing, mingling, and conversing with other partygoers till the wee hours. Unless the party-giver is a vegetarian, you'll have protein for dinner, so breakfast should include hot or cold cereal or an egg. If you choose the egg, have a salad or soup for lunch, and if you choose the cereal for breakfast, have an egg for lunch. If you think you're hungry before you're ready to leave for the party, have a Fourth Meal of a little cold cereal, or an egg, if you haven't had that item previously that day. Ascertain whether a protein or a nonprotein meal would be appropriate. This should take the edge off your hunger.

Recommit to three goals.

1. Remember your ultimate weight-loss goal and think: "I want to weigh _____ pounds."

2. Plan, in writing, the categories of foods you're going to eat (do you need a protein or nonprotein meal?); the number of items (is the meal to contain one item? Two items? Three or more?); Filler or not, and if so, which one.

3. If the plan isn't working, know what you're going to do with repatterning, so when you arrive at the party and the Swedish meatball says *ya,* you'll be prepared with a *na.*

Are you nervous or anxious? There are a lot of new people to meet. You might even be tired, tense, or bored. But if you take my pre-party advice and eat wisely before you leave your home, you probably will not be hungry during the cocktail hour. This is a perfect moment to fill up another glass of water. Now walk around. Introduce yourself to those you don't know. Offer an extra pair of hands to the father of the bride, or maybe chat with a neglected grandmother. If it is not a family function and you're single, flirt with others or talk to the person in the cowboy hat and convince him or her you adore country music.

A difficult moment? A tray come too close? Take a deep breath. Yes, it does look good, but it's not a reason to eat. Yes, it does smell good, but it's not a reason to eat. Yes, you might be anxious, but it's not a reason to eat. And besides, you want to weigh _____ pounds. There may be many other moments to get through, including Karen and Kevin Koaxer. They insist you eat whatever they eat, and they opt for everything in sight. They actually try to put food into your mouth, all the while saying, "Taste this. Try that!" These people are pushers, and you want to push away from them as quickly as possible. "Excuse me. I see someone over there and I want to say hello."

Your first attempt at following your plan could be a little awkward— not as comfortable as the old way. You might be feeling withdrawal symptoms from the excessive eating you've practiced and perfected at parties for decades. But being stuffed and bloated at the bash is far more uncomfortable than changing a few habits tonight. And besides,

- No one cares what you eat or drink.

- No one knows you're trying to change your habits.

- No one will stop inviting you to their parties because you didn't overeat at this one.

- The invitation in your pocket or purse tells you dinner is imminent.

- Your hostess or host only wants you to have a good time. Walk. Talk. Cha-cha-cha.

The Best Man begins an evening of toasts. The music swells as you find your place cards and sit down.

And, now for dinner—and the next hurdles. Bread sticks stand in silver cups, and butter is served in squat-footed dishes. Fruit compote is nestled in a glass bowl on crushed ice. The centerpiece contains pale pink peonies intertwined with roses that match the tablecloths and napkins. Everything is elegant and beautiful.

My Thinking

Bread sticks are commonplace. Fruit compote is dessert on your program, and besides, you're opting for a piece of wedding cake. The salad course is nothing special, and the dressing has limped the lettuce. No, thank you. Cold potato soup looks interesting, but soup is often an entire meal, so you decline that too. During the bread, fruit compote, salad, and soup courses, dance. Drink water. Talk to the person seated next to you. If you are not eating, move.

The main course is perfectly prepared prime rib and delectable duckling, parsley potatoes, and an interesting carrot concoction. Some celebrants ask for a little of each. It's easier to watch your portion size if you select the rib *or* duckling, plus the potatoes, and the carrots. Delicious.

Cousins kissing over there. An old friend spots you and dances toward you to visit. You hug as you glide along the perimeter of the room playing, "Did you see so and so?"

Cookies and pastries arrive and look interesting, but wedding cake, which looks even more delectable, is part of your original plan. While you're waiting, dance with the bride or groom.

Recommit to your goals. The first goal is how much you want to weigh; the next goal is what you want to accomplish at this function. Continue toasting with water. Thank the waiter for delivering your piece of wedding cake with extra butter-cream flowers piled on top. Yumm.

The party favors are little silver baskets filled with miniature candies. You keep the silver basket, with details of the event engraved on the side, and leave the sweets on the table. This is no time to think you can handle it. And besides, you've had dessert in the form of wedding cake.

A singer is entertaining with a sentimental "Sunrise, Sunset." There's not a dry eye in the house.

The bouquet is tossed. The garter goes to an usher. The flower girl falls asleep in her mother's lap. The four-year-old ring bearer doesn't understand why he doesn't get to keep the ring and crawls under a table in protest.

As you exit, the harpist and cellist are playing "The Party's Over." Because your clothing still feels loose, you won't have to open the zipper on your pants or dress on the way home. And I'll bet you feel even better because you planned what to do and did it. When you arrive home, you're not as terribly uncomfortable as you usually are after these affairs, you don't stay up all night with indigestion, and there won't be a need to berate yourself the following morning for eating too much because you didn't. You simply planned ahead, went, had a wonderful time, and food was but a part of it all.

And your friend or relative got married, and they did it without your overeating. Imagine that.

Holiday Eating Strategy Review

Almost every month has a holiday where food is the centerpiece. The holiday eating strategies are helpful if you read the information before, during, and after the festivities. This will help you plan ahead, execute, evaluate, and adjust, for next time. That's the thing with holidays—there's always a next time.

**I want to weigh _____ pounds, 365 days a year,
not just when it's convenient.**

Holiday Eating Strategies
- Don't skip meals. Starving all day as an excuse to overeat at a party doesn't work. Plan ahead instead.

- In a relaxed, quiet atmosphere, envision what food and drink you'll be encountering and plan, in advance, *in writing,* what you want to do. How many items are appropriate? What are they to be? Chicken? Fish? Veal? Will you choose a potato? What behavioral techniques do you plan to use to help lessen food-related anxiety?

- Wear a belt with a buckle, whenever eating and whenever necessary. Buckle on snug. Wear a thin belt under your clothes if the outfit is of the cover-up variety.

- While in attendance, keep moving. Help the hostess, play with children, and talk to everyone in the room before looking at the food. Don't linger near the buffet table.

- Fill a glass with water. Carry it around, and drink it. Throughout the party and whenever necessary, relax, deep-breathe, and stretch to reduce socially anxious moments. If wall-to-wall food is a given, consider arriving a little late.

- If it is a buffet meal, make yourself a plate as you might be served in a restaurant. Plan the number of items in advance. Decide, before arriving, whether you'll choose a bread *or* beverage *or* dessert *or* alcohol rather than deciding you'll have all four. (Is the bread really unique, the coffee unusual, the extra drink adding to your enjoyment?)

- Find a place to eat where you can enjoy your meal in a relaxed manner while using utensils. If this is not possible or the choices are really not to your liking, consider leaving early.

- It is okay to tell your hosts you don't want a second helping of everything. They only want you to have a good time. You won't be having a good time if you eat too much and your clothes become tight. Overeating is not a reward. Fill up on the ambiance.

- Eat slowly and thoughtfully. Make each meal last a relaxing 20 minutes or more. Put down your utensils, take frequent sips of water, and intersperse plenty of good conversation between bites.

- Alcohol causes lack of resolve, which may cause you to eat or drink too much of things you didn't plan for. Less and less alcohol is needed as your total body weight diminishes. If alcohol is your choice instead of bread, beverage, or dessert, toast the holiday, but try to drink two sips or more of water for each sip of alcohol. And bear in mind, nobody said you have to finish your drink.

- Remember, there will always be another meal, another holiday, another party. Keep in mind how much more fun they will be with a slimmer waistline.

- Do the best you can. There are a lot of choices to make. The first time, your plan may not turn out exactly as you pictured it to be. By reading your strategies and planning in advance, in writing, what you want to accomplish, chances are you'll eat a little less, move a little more, put your fork down sooner, and feel a little better than had you not had a plan. But, no matter what happens, *get back on The Program at the very next meal.*

- Most of all, have a nice time. Feeling stuffed, bloated, or uncomfortable in your clothes does not enhance the enjoyment of the event. More is not better; it is only more.

- Rewrite these *Holiday Eating Strategies* onto a compact piece of paper. Carry it with you to read before and during the party. Repeat your goals to yourself several times during the day of the food encounter. When you're sufficiently armed, the battle is won.

- If all else fails, flee the city with a friend.

Cruise Ship or Resort

The - unlimited - quantity - all - you - can - eat - comes - with - the - room - vacation—whether on a cruise ship or at a resort—is an American classic experience, but forget "you may never pass this way again" and think, instead: "I want to weigh _____ pounds!" The everything-included vacation is here to challenge you.

My own experience was not on the high seas but in the mountains. Having spent my first seventeen years in the Catskills as the second daughter of hotel people, I was familiar with Jewish-style cooking, abundant portions, and a wide variety of food choices. There were also the unlimited appetizers, entrées, side orders, and desserts, all for the price of a night's stay in a hotel.

Years later, I find myself conducting two weight-control workshops at the now-defunct, and legendary, Concord Hotel.

Could a single encounter with the hotel dining room undo years of wonderful eating habits? Hardly. Was it easy? Easier than imagined, but I had a plan.

Thinking about the weekend in advance, I pack my lightweight scale and a logbook in which to take notes. Since I have a solid foundation of experience about which foods work for me, I only have to find them in the book of foods the hotel jokingly refers to as a menu. In addition to knowing which foods I want, I also have a clear vision of how many items allow me to maintain my weight each day. And, of course I know my portion size.

You can assume there will be many more items than you normally serve yourself, and you can assume the portion size and unlimited choices will also be greater than you'd ever purchase or prepare at home. Within these guidelines however, there is wonderful leeway if you remember you cannot possibly eat it all, and it is not the last meal you'll ever eat. Just because the hotel promotes unlimited everything is no reason to have six desserts and three entrées.

Unlimited portions equal an unlimited body.

If you have difficulty connecting your feelings of physical discomfort with the all-you-can-eat food policy of the hotel, you're probably not thinking that a consequence comes with every mouthful.

When I arrive at 11:00 p.m., a free dinner pass to the coffee shop is attached to my registration card. Scribbled on it in red pencil are the words *late arrival.* The coffee shop needs study, but having eaten before I left my apartment, I'm not hungry.

The menu contains many sandwiches, pancakes, waffles, desserts, and a full soda fountain. There are also bagels, lox, cream cheese, and all possible variations on a theme, plus several varieties of omelets. There are no vegetables, salads, soup, or protein alone on the menu. These items are only offered with a sandwich or some other food. I walk to the nightclub.

Tom Jones is the guest singer. The club waiter brings me the water I request. There is no pushing of alcohol.

Harriet E. asks what to do if not having a drink is an issue. I tell her that I used to go to a comedy club where there was a two-drink minimum. My friends and I would arrive after dinner. I would order water. If my friends didn't want the two drinks I had paid for anyway, I'd send my drinks to an adjoining table. I considered it all part of the cost of entertainment. Every situation is different.

If someone insists you have a drink, have at the ready the right words to firmly refuse the drink (or food). You might say you have to be up early or you have an appointment and can't be fuzzy. Maybe you're taking an antibiotic and shouldn't be drinking alcohol. Be creative because you want to weigh _____ pounds. It is no one's business but your own whether you have a drink. Maybe you've been clean and sober for years. *No* is *no* in any language.

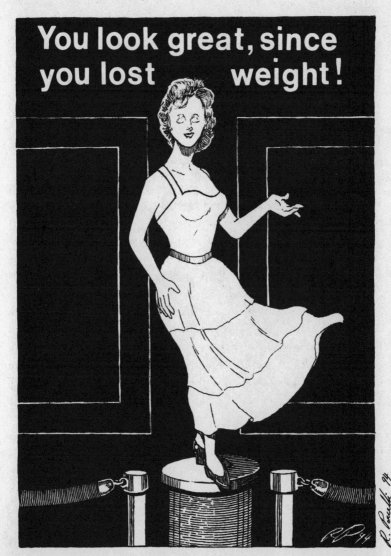

After the show, the lounge poses no problem either. I ask for and receive a glass of water, talk with a few people, and go to my room.

Morning brings *breakfast is being served in the main dining room.* Let the food for the day begin. Baskets of bread, rolls, muffins, and bagels appear on the table. Separate platters of butter and cheese spreads clus-

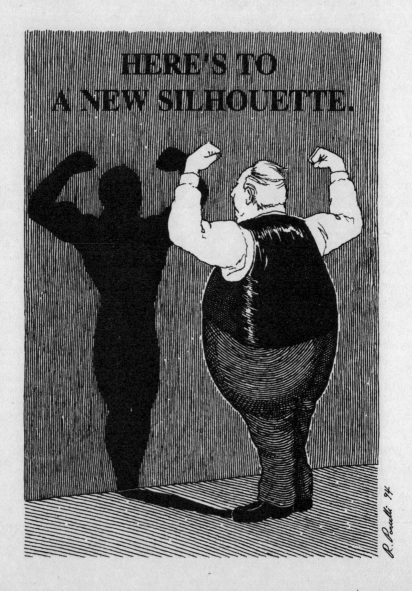

ter nearby. A steaming pitcher of coffee is set next to me. The menu contains a surprisingly comprehensive offering of hot and cold cereals, eggs any style with or without onions, lox, and whatever is usual, plus fruits and fruit juices.

I opt for hot cereal and a cup of hot water. After 20 minutes of filling up on the conversation at the table and watching the man next to me finish his second basket of bread, I am not hungry any more. Just as I am leaving the table, a busboy clears my plate, and a waiter comes to ask for my egg order. No, thank you, I smile; I'm fine. And I am.

Yes, there are a lot of interesting things on the menu, but to be perfectly honest, if you've tasted one miniature Danish at breakfast, you've tasted them all. I enjoy my oatmeal at home, and it never occurs to me to eat an egg with it. A bowl of cereal is enough at home, and it is enough while in a hotel. Enough is enough no matter which way you slice it.

I walk the extensive and beautiful grounds of the hotel while exploring the options for physical activity. There is an indoor and an outdoor pool; a weight room, steam room, and sauna; aerobics; massage; cards to play; Ping-Pong, shuffleboard, dance lessons, tennis, horseback riding, and, in the winter, skiing. I opt for Ping-Pong and get an unexpected workout—my partner is a very competitive tri-athlete. Before I know it, lunch is being served.

I choose cold poached fish. Although I could have several main courses—per the unlimited-quantity-of-food policy of the hotel—I ask instead for one potato pancake with my fish. Both singular portions prove to be enormous. The potato pancake is served with applesauce and sour cream. I choose neither. The pancake is delicious by itself.

There's a four o'clock buffet, but I'm finally winning at Ping-Pong. I'm not hungry anyway. Dinner is uneventful, and, during the midnight buffet, I watch a dance exhibition.

The rest of the evening I spend walking, sitting, dancing, speaking with others, and eventually watching the show.

Here are some things you can do when on your next vacation or trip:

- Know, in writing, what you are trying to accomplish at each meal before you sit down to eat.

- Know the number of items you are going to eat before you order them.

- Think how much greater the portion size is than what you serve yourself at home.

- Slow down, deep-breathe, and refresh yourself before eating.

- Imagine that Chef Murray weighs 350 pounds, and *his* portion size is on your plate. Leave some food on the plate.

If you make choices before, during, and after each meal, you'll have sampled a variety of different foods, and won't have gained any weight. You might have even lost a few pounds.

Think of a cruise as a floating hotel. If you're considering a spa, don't let the illusion of healthy food and physical activity trick you into eating when you're not hungry or eating more than you need, just because you did a few leg lifts. The same guidelines prevail.

Bon voyage.

The Beginning

Congratulations. You completed the book—the basics of The Program. You have some of the tools, but not all. That comes with experience. That comes with familiarity about how The Program works. That comes with practice.

The memory is short. You've changed. You're a different person than you were two days, two weeks, two months ago. Go back to the beginning of the book, and begin reading it again.

As the concepts of The Program become comfortable, you almost forget that a scant few weeks ago, you weren't doing any of the things you now do. As the scale goes onward and downward, don't get cocky, complacent, or too comfortable so you begin to think you don't have to do the assignments anymore. You do. I do. We all do.

One of my favorite movies is *Groundhog Day* starring Bill Murray. In the movie, he portrays a man who keeps reliving Groundhog Day over and over. It is Mr. Murray's genius that he changed each day in small, incremental, subtle ways. Some changes might not have been noticed, but he changed.

1. He planned.

2. He executed.

3. He evaluated, and

4. He adjusted.

He achieved his goal: he got the girl.

You'll do the same four things he did and achieve your goal of weighing _____ pounds.

Let me hear an *I can do it!*

Let me hear an *I did it and I'm proud!*

Let me hear an *I know what I did, and I'll do it again and again.* When you do The Program, it works. When you stop doing The Program, it stops working.

Extract the meat and potatoes from The Program. Take time to digest it all. When you do, it is all the sweeter because you did it yourself.

Now, go back to the beginning and begin again.

Acknowledgments

There are many people to acknowledge. Some of them helped me get through the day so I could write; some helped me in ways of which they're not even aware. Some encouraged me to stay in business when it didn't look as if I should; some lent money to me to keep me afloat when I was sinking and broke; some even called to make sure my phone was working. Many took a chance on my program, the behavioral approach to weight loss on which this book is based. Still more referred their friends. Everyone encouraged me to continue writing.

Where I've used initials (scrambled or otherwise), it was to thank someone who might not want their name in a book about conquering food addiction. I respect that.

I want to thank N.R., Ph.D., the first person ever to go through The Program on April 11, 1981. He continued to have faith in The Program and continued to send people until he moved out of state. What a wonderful beginning.

I am grateful to the late Brent Collins, a friend who was an actor as well as a book producer for a large publishing house. When I started out many years ago, he gave me as much freelance typing work as I needed to support myself while launching the initial stages of The Program. He innocently suggested that if I wrote a book, he'd be happy to show it to people he knew in the industry.

Thanks to the late Jeff Dames, my dear dear friend, for encouraging my writing since we were children together. He typed an early incarnation of the book with fun margin notes when all we had were electric typewriters, carbon paper, and correction fluid.

Thanks to my friend Lindy Laher Pomerantz, who not only encouraged my writing but saved it. I value her comments about some sentences, paragraphs, and chapters in the book. But mostly I value her friendship.

To my friend Joan Lefkowitz, for helping me set monthly goals for business and life and by being at the other end of the phone to help me get over the humps and bumps on the road to having a successful business and being a more successful me.

To my friend Charlie Kaye, for helping me get through ups and downs, illnesses and health, successes and failures. He is always there with a professional eye and a humorist's heart.

To Linda Morel, a writer friend who would sign off on her notes to me: *Keep writing.*

Thanks to Gerri Baum, a writer friend who also encouraged me to keep writing. I especially loved how she'd scribble the words *great* and *wonderful* at the top of a page, then gently suggest what might make it tighter or more crisp, or how to make a point better. She was always right.

And thanks to all program participants whose stories fill the book. To all the sharing and insights and perseverance, determination, and amazement when they realize they could lose weight after a two-birthday-party week, as well as over a four-day Fourth of July weekend.

To one of Gotham Writer's nonfiction Tuesday night groups, whose input was varied and wonderful. A special nod to the teacher Deborah Emin, for her constructive comments, though I couldn't always read her handwriting. Thanks to Allison Tyler, who continued to read chapters at Tuesday night get-togethers in my apartment. She was always of good cheer and positivity, and thoughtful in her remarks.

To my friend Risa Starr, who introduced me to Deb Futter, an editor for a major publisher.

And thanks to Deb Futter who when I said, "The book is ready and I'm ready," introduced me to Esther Newberg, my agent at ICM. Thanks to Esther Newberg for sending my book to precisely the right person who became my editor, Fred Hills. And thanks to Fred for believing in my message and my work, and for buying the book.

Thanks to Carolyn Nakano, the person who typed the manuscript many times with never-ending support and patience. She brought charts and illustrations to life as well as a calming serenity to my home office.

Thanks to Sy Safransky, for allowing me to see my name in print many times in his Reader's Write Section of his little gem of a magazine, *The Sun.*

Thanks to Rick Dames, Harvard Tigler, David Grant, Robert Chiu, and Dianne Rooney for being there for me when I needed them.

Thank you, Loretta Denner, for your thorough and patient helpfulness.

And thanks to everyone who never once in twenty years asked: "Are you *still* writing that book?"

Index